T0043086

TUNING
the
Human
Biofield

"*Tuning the Human Biofield* is a superb introduction to the human energy field and its modification by sound vibrations. McKusick's book is a highly valuable resource for patients and practitioners alike."

GARY E. SCHWARTZ, PH.D., PROFESSOR OF PSYCHOLOGY, MEDICINE, NEUROLOGY, PSYCHIATRY, AND SURGERY AT THE UNIVERSITY OF ARIZONA AND AUTHOR OF *THE LIVING ENERGY UNIVERSE* AND *THE ENERGY HEALING EXPERIMENTS*

"This book takes the reader by the hand on a quick tour through the 'wonderland' of quantum theory, vibrational therapies, the electric universe, biofield science, and other frontier science topics. Autobiographical bits and pieces make for enjoyable and easy reading. . . . a promising modality to reduce stress and improve energy flow toward greater wellness."

BEVERLY RUBIK, PH.D., PROFESSOR AT ENERGY MEDICINE UNIVERSITY AND PRESIDENT/FOUNDER OF THE INSTITUTE FOR FRONTIER SCIENCE

"This book integrates core universal truths with scientific principles to capture the essence of sound healing. As a pioneer in the field of sound healing, the author combines her knowledge, expertise, curiosity, and unique personal experience into an easy-to-learn method that can offer powerful changes for the reader."

MELISSA JOY JONSSON, PRESIDENT/INSTRUCTOR AT MATRIX ENERGETICS INTERNATIONAL AND AUTHOR OF *M-JOY PRACTICALLY SPEAKING: MATRIX ENERGETICS* AND *LIVING YOUR INFINITE POTENTIAL*

"The time has come for detailed explorations by skilled, sensitive, and intuitive individuals who are willing to venture into the unknown, to go beyond the mainstream and report on the discoveries they make. Eileen McKusick has all of the tools such an explorer requires, including a skeptical and scientific grounding. Enjoy this feast of new knowledge—it is guaranteed to stick to your ribs!"

JAMES L. OSCHMAN, PH.D., AUTHOR OF
ENERGY MEDICINE: THE SCIENTIFIC BASIS

"An excellent explanation of how the tuning forks can influence the subtle fields for healing. Thought-provoking and detailed in explanation, this book is also an excellent reference guide to using the tuning forks in a treatment mode for the various chakra energy centers. A must-read for anyone thinking of using tuning forks as a healing tool."

JEFFREY THOMPSON, D.C.,
CENTER FOR NEUROACOUSTIC RESEARCH

"Eileen Day McKusick has meticulously gathered biofield research that supports the efficacy of Biofield Tuning. *Tuning the Human Biofield* is comprehensive yet easy to read. With this, sound-on-body becomes understandable and practical for health-care professionals and individual self-healing."

JOSHUA LEEDS, AUTHOR OF
THE POWER OF SOUND AND *THROUGH A DOG'S EAR*

"*Tuning the Human Biofield* is a profoundly insightful and inspiring work as well as a tremendous leap forward for the healing sciences. If I were designing an alternative medicine curriculum, this text would be required reading. In what is arguably the most comprehensive book ever written on tuning fork therapy, Eileen Day McKusick not only shows us the door to healing ourselves and unlocking our potential as energetic beings, she also takes us by the hand and, brilliantly and eloquently, escorts us into new realms of possibility."

SOL LUCKMAN, AUTHOR OF
CONSCIOUS HEALING AND *POTENTIATE YOUR DNA*

"McKusick's audacity and confidence coupled with her serious, in-depth research and humility puts her at the forefront of cutting-edge science and healing. This book explains and enlivens our understanding of interconnectivity and consciousness and helps us deeply understand how we humans function, and how we can function better."

LAUREN WALKER, AUTHOR OF *ENERGY MEDICINE YOGA*

TUNING
the
Human
Biofield

Healing with
Vibrational
Sound Therapy

Eileen Day McKusick

Healing Arts Press
One Park Street
Rochester, Vermont 05767
www.HealingArtsPress.com

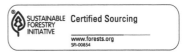

Text stock is SFI certified

Healing Arts Press is a division of Inner Traditions International

Copyright © 2014, 2021 by Eileen Day McKusick
Foreword copyright © 2014, 2021 by Karl H. Maret, M.D.

All rights reserved. No part of this book may be reproduced or utilized in
any form or by any means, electronic or mechanical, including photocopying,
recording, or by any information storage and retrieval system, without permission
in writing from the publisher.

Note to the reader: This book is intended as an informational guide. The
remedies, approaches, and techniques described herein are meant to supplement,
and not to be a substitute for, professional medical care or treatment. They should
not be used to treat a serious ailment without prior consultation with a qualified
health care professional.

Cataloging-in-Publication Data for this title is available from the Library of Congress

ISBN 978-1-64411-318-9 (print)
ISBN 978-1-64411-319-6 (ebook)

Printed and bound in the United States by Lake Book Manufacturing, Inc.
The text stock is SFI certified. The Sustainable Forestry Initiative® program
promotes sustainable forest management.

10 9 8 7 6 5 4

Text design by Virginia Scott Bowman

This book was typeset in Garamond Premier Pro with Eurostile used as the
display typeface

To send correspondence to the author of this book, mail a first-class letter to the
author c/o Inner Traditions • Bear & Company, One Park Street, Rochester, VT
05767, and we will forward the communication, or contact the author directly at
www.eileenmckusick.com.

CONTENTS

BIOFIELD TUNING REFINED

In 2015, shortly after this book was written, I had the inspiration to change the name of the sound therapy method that I was then calling sound balancing to Biofield Tuning. In the first edition of this book, the practice is referred to throughout by the former term; in this edition it has been changed to reflect the new name.

Sound balancing refers to the general idea that sound can be used to balance the tonal outputs of the body. We can do sound balancing with any instrument, including tuning forks, gongs, bowls, bells, cellos, drums, and more. However, Biofield Tuning is a very specific approach with a very detailed manual, the official practice of which requires training and certification.

Readers of this book are welcome to use the approach shared here with friends and family, and those who already have an established professional practice are also welcome to incorporate these ideas into their practice. However, the information contained in this book is not sufficient to call what you are doing Biofield Tuning, as that term is reserved for certified practitioners only.

Additionally, the approach to the method has also changed, and as a result the "Getting Started with the Forks" chapter has been considerably rewritten in this edition.

June 1, 2020

FOREWORD

KARL H. MARET, M.D.

This book by Eileen McKusick is a little gem, a valuable contribution to the field of sound healing and energy medicine. The author is a courageous pioneer in the emerging field of biofield science investigating the effects of tuning forks on the human energetic anatomy. It is also the very personal story of a searcher for truth, understanding, and synthesis at the frontiers of healing.

I first met Eileen in 2011 when she asked me to review her thesis for her master of education degree. This led to meeting her in person in the fall of that year. I found her to be scientifically astute, with an inquiring mind, a well-functioning intuition, and an unusually well-developed sense of clairaudience, allowing her to hear and discern seeming imbalances in the biofield around human beings. To her credit, she sought to discover the significance of her unconventional observations in a scientifically grounded manner with a great deal of discernment, as you will discover while reading this book. Hers is a story of discovery leading from original observations gained through working with people suffering from various afflictions, to the search for an understanding and explanation of her unique perceptions. Some of these stories are recounted in this book. It appears that she has been able to share her unique gifts with a growing number of students who are now also applying this new sound healing approach with their clients.

I have personally experienced the power of her healing approach with tuning forks and recognized early on that this method deserved further scientific investigation. When she worked with a number of clients at our clinic in California, she was able to make profound changes in their physiology as evidenced by a lessening of pain, greater mobility, and a sense of deep relaxation and well-being. One of my clients reported after an hour-long session of biofield therapy with Eileen, "It felt as if a weight had been taken off my shoulders." Most clients were surprised at the level of detail that Eileen was able to perceive about their past history and the trauma patterns held in their body. It appears that the body's biofield either "stores" or has access to historical information that was encoded over a lifetime of experiences. If these sound healing approaches can be verified with further scientific studies, a new healing paradigm may be imminent.

In 1962 Thomas Kuhn published the book *The Structure of Scientific Revolutions* making the scientific community aware of the nature of paradigm shifts. A paradigm serves as a pattern or model of existing beliefs that anchors consensual reality. A prominent paradigm in contemporary medicine is that we are primarily biochemical beings. Under this established paradigm, a whole pharmaceutical industry has emerged that essentially dictates that drugs are one of the most effective approaches to bring about symptom modulation and (hopefully) healing in an organism. This paradigm is now beginning to be questioned by increasing numbers of practitioners and patients alike.

Over the last three decades a new paradigm has been emerging—that we are more fundamentally energetic and informational beings with sophisticated, high-speed communication channels in our living connective tissue matrix, capable of rapidly affecting tissues, cellular processes, and even nuclear DNA expression. These processes are better described using the language and principles of quantum physics, including quantum resonance, entanglement, and nonlocality or action-at-a-distance, which is beginning to be applied to macroscopic processes inside living organisms. This new physics describes a world that appears increasingly paradoxical, counterintuitive, and confusing to our fundamental sense perceptions. Our current medicine does not utilize these concepts, but rather relies on classical Newtonian physics and Lucretian biochemistry. From this more deterministic and materialistic perspective, modern medical science would view the idea of healing with tuning forks as outlined in this book with considerable skepticism.

Nonetheless, it is now well accepted that we live in an invisible ocean of energy-suffusing space. The 2013 Nobel Prize in physics was won by Peter Higgs and François Englert for their theoretical discovery of a mechanism that contributes to our understanding of the origins of mass and diversity in the universe. This was recently confirmed through the discovery of the predicted fundamental particle called the Higgs boson at CERN's Large Hadron Collider in Geneva. What today's cutting-edge physicists are showing is that we exist in an ocean of potentiality and latent energy that is present in the quantum vacuum, or in reality the quantum plenum, the sea of almost infinite energy in which matter and mass manifest and disappear continuously. All manifestation, including our bodies, is immersed in this invisible energetic ocean. Ultimately, we interact through quantum physical processes with these energetic fields that are embedded within space-time. Concepts of healing energy that were once viewed with suspicion and even ridicule are now beginning to gain respectability and are becoming the subject of active investigation.

One of the main reasons for this change in outlook is that sensitive electromagnetic instruments have been developed that are capable of detecting minute energy fields around the human body. One of these is the SQUID (superconducting quantum interference device) magnetometer capable of detecting tiny biomagnetic fields associated with physiological activities occurring within the body. This is the same field that sensitive individuals have described for thousands of years, which was formerly ignored by scientists because there had been no objective way to measure it.

For over one hundred years, scientists have shown that cells and tissues generate electrical fields that can be measured on the surface of the skin. All cells generate tiny electrical currents as a result of charge flow that makes life possible. Electrical currents in turn generate tiny magnetic fields in the surrounding space. The electrocardiogram, measured from electrodes placed on the surface of the body, informs clinicians about the electrical activities of the heart. Even smaller currents and potentials are picked up around our head with an electroencephalogram (EEG). In specially shielded rooms, using the SQUID technologies described above, scientists can also record the tiny magnetic fields originating in the brain or the heart at some distance from the body. These are called the magnetoencephalogram and magnetocardiogram, respectively. It is quite likely that in the future scientists will study the effect of sound fields on the body using such sophisticated instruments to gain further insights into the pioneering discoveries described in this book.

We now know that all tissues and organs produce specific magnetic pulsations that collectively are called biomagnetic fields. Mapping the magnetic fields in the space around the body often provides a more accurate indication of physiological and pathological states compared to more traditional electrical field measurements on the surface of the body. For example, in the 1980s Dr. John Zimmerman, then at the University of Colorado's School of Medicine, used SQUID magnetometers to measure the pulsing biomagnetic field emanating from the hands of therapeutic touch practitioners. He found that these energy healers produced frequencies of pulsations that literally swept between 0.3 and 30 Hertz (cycles per second), the same extremely low-frequency (ELF) range in which the brain operates. These same frequencies are capable of creating powerful healing responses in any part of the body.

This work was confirmed in 1992 by Seto and colleagues in Japan, who studied "Qi emissions" in practitioners of various martial arts and healing methods, using magnetometers consisting of two coils of wire with 80,000 turns. Since then there have been further studies extending these investigations to sound, light, and thermal fields emitted by qigong practitioners. Specific frequencies stimulate the growth of nerves, bones, blood capillaries, ligaments, connective tissue, and skin. Orthopedic surgeons have used low-level magnetic bone stimulators for several decades to heal nonunion fractures in bones.

Although we have known about brain waves since 1929 as a result of the pioneering work of German psychiatrist Hans Berger that led to the discovery of the electroencephalograph, we now know that these low-frequency waves are not confined only to the brain, but actually spread throughout the body via the perineural system, the connective tissue sheaths that surround all nerves. The late Dr. Robert Becker has described this system as regulating injury repair processes throughout the body.[1] From this perspective one can visualize the entire nervous system as a giant antenna that both perceives and even projects biomagnetic pulsations throughout the body and into the body's biofield. The perineural system is embedded within the entire living matrix, the energetic communication system within the body.

The origin of the concept of the living matrix goes back to Claude Bernard, one of the nineteenth-century physiology pioneers, who coined the term *le milieu intérieur,* or "the interior environment of the body." Bernard did not believe in the idea of vital energy and sought to describe physiological regulation and communication strictly in biochemical and biophysical terms. He introduced the concept of *homeostasis,* a term that was actually coined in 1926 by Walter Cannon, referring to the inner regulatory capacity of the body that ensures a stable environment for the tissues and organs.

Further research into the energetic aspects of this interior communication system was carried out by Nobel laureate Albert Szent-Györgyi. He concluded that organic communication could not be explained solely by the random collision of molecules and purely chemical processes. As early as 1941 he described quantum physical and bioenergetics processes accompanying complex regulation within the connective tissue matrix through electrons and protons flowing as charge transference along hydrated proteins acting as semiconductors. This idea was initially received with skepticism, but it is now generally accepted that most, if not all, parts of the extracellular matrix have semiconductor properties. This makes the living matrix appear as a complex information-processing system analogous to modern computer chips, only vastly more complex.

In the 1950s Dr. Szent-Györgyi laid out the theory of bioenergetics, in which he described how energy can flow through electromagnetic fields inside living organisms, which, as a result of the ubiquitous nature of water inside the organism, forms the matrix of life. He wrote, "The transmission of excitation energies between molecules through electromagnetic coupling is not a mere matter of speculation."[2] These energies flow through water channels inside the body, since over 99 percent of the molecules inside the body are water molecules and the body is two-thirds water by volume. Every protein, whether constituting bone, sinews, or any other tissue, exists in a hydrated form. When the water content of the body decreases to less than 50 percent, we die. Protons and electrons separate along membranes to create charged layers analogous to a tiny battery, as the revolutionary work of Gerald Pollack at the University of Washington has recently shown.[3] In this inner electrical environment of our bodies, the magic of life unfolds, and this environment can also be influenced in a powerful manner through sound vibrations.

In the past medical students were taught that biochemical interactions are the basis of life, and that molecules fitting into receptors trigger cellular responses, both inside and outside the cells. Yet scientists like Szent-Györgyi, Jim Oschman, and Dr. Albrecht-Buehler have pointed out that life processes are too fast to be explained by molecules wandering around and diffusing in and out of cells.[4] Instead, molecules interact through electromagnetic resonances very similar to tuning forks or pendulum clocks that begin to oscillate in unison through resonance processes. Resonance phenomena occur with many types of vibration and in all kinds of media. Tissues have mechanical, acoustic, electrical, and magnetic resonances, to name just a few. Nuclear magnetic resonances are used medically to excite hydrogen atoms inside the water of the body to create visible resonance pictures of one's internal anatomy for diagnostic purposes.

Everything in the universe is in vibration. The science of spectroscopy allows us to characterize atoms and molecules through the emissions and absorptions of different electromagnetic waves, including visible and invisible light. When electrons in molecules vibrate, they produce electromagnetic fields that depend on their frequency and on the ways they interact with their neighboring electrons and nearby molecules. Chemists use spectra to identify elements, while biophysicists use them to describe the molecular interactions inside cells and tissues.

The work of the late Ross Adey showed that there are specific resonance windows in which biological effects tend to take place preferentially. Biological cellular reactions take place at just the right frequency and amplitude, often at very low intensities. Too powerful a signal might not create a biological response, but a tiny signal at just the right frequency is capable of triggering cell membrane proteins to create an amplified response inside a cell or its DNA genetic material.[5] It is thus not surprising that the subtle energetic emanations from a tuning fork at a specific resonant frequency could have an unforeseen healing effect on the body.

It is also important to differentiate between energy and information, or literally, subtle energy. Information is patterned energy that can be carried by electromagnetic waves modulated in different ways. Consider a television receiver that is connected to an antenna on the roof. We can take a sensitive detecting device called a spectrum analyzer and measure a whole range of different frequencies as well as their various intensities over time. However, simply measuring these energy or field intensities does not allow you to know very much about the data or information content carried on these electromagnetic waves. To understand how this information reappears as a television picture you need to know the unique algorithms used at the transmitting station to originally encode the information. Once you unscramble or decode this information inside the receiver, you can learn whether a certain channel contained a news program, a drama presentation, or a sports event. The information is what's important to the viewer, even though the electromagnetic resonances or carrier waves are necessary to carry the data to the appropriately tuned receiver. The body works in a similar manner: it is able to decode complex streams of environmental information that can lead to health or disease. The human genetic code or genome, which is present in almost every cell of our bodies, can be activated by environmental signals through a process of epigenetic signaling.

Most people think of sound transmitted through the air as a succession of longitudinal pressure waves passed along by the molecules of air that show alternating areas of compression and rarefaction. A microphone is a simple transducer that translates pressure waves into electrical signals that can be amplified and reproduced through a loudspeaker. However, this view of sound waves is deceptive because sound is propagated through spherical wave fronts expanding as a series of concentric bubbles from the sound source. Viewed from this perspective, sound is analogous to electromagnetic waves, which also expand as spherical fields but travel much faster, at the speed of light (300 million meters per second), compared to the much slower speed of propagation of sound in air (around 343 meters per second or 1234.37 kilometers per hour).

In water and watery solids such as the human body, sound travels over four times faster, in the form of phonons, or sonic shear waves. As the sound emanating from tuning forks strikes the body's skin interface, complex electrical and phonon interactions take place that can alter tissue dielectric properties, including various acupuncture meridians. The meridians have different electrical properties than their surrounding tissue. Thus, when a holographic sound field such as that produced by a tuning fork, which contains complex data structures of pure frequencies with changing phase relationships, strikes the biofield of a person, the cellular memories of various tissues can be reawakened, potentially leading to a healing response. Quantum physical field theory predicts the occurrence of a number of coherent dynamic phenomena in liquid water inside cells and tissues that may be stimulated by sound. This process affects the free electron clouds existing within these coherent water domains.[6] Thus sound will interact with membrane regions called watery exclusion zones (or EZ layers) that can in turn modify cellular processes through their interaction with the hydration shells surrounding cell membrane receptors.

Quantum physics applied to living systems is not a new concept.

One of the earliest pioneers was Herbert Fröhlich, who suggested that quantum coherence existed in living systems. Several groups working with him helped to elucidate that liquid crystalline components of the body can produce Bose-Einstein condensation of strongly excited longitudinal electric modes, long-range coherence, and energy storage inside cells and tissues.[7] This allows for biological responses to extremely weak electromagnetic fields, including subtle energetic interactions with the environment. Recently, a new generation of quantum physicists has developed the self-field theory (SFT), applying new models of expanded quantum physics to biological molecules and biological evolution. The fields in SFT are discrete streams of photons with an internal bispinoral structure rather than the continuous fields of Maxwell's classical electrodynamics.[8] In this new model of the photon, the force carrier in electromagnetism, there are three types of interactions with matter, namely, electric, magnetic, and acoustic. From this vantage point, new explanations of acoustic interactions with matter might soon lead to a more acceptable theoretical foundation of the biophysics of sound healing. These approaches have already been applied successfully to healing with sound in animals.[9]

The Eastern yogic sciences have a long history of incorporating models of consciousness into their descriptions of the nature of reality. Western science only began actively addressing the issue of consciousness and the observer effect in quantum mechanics during the twentieth century. This new physics has changed our whole view of reality by incorporating consciousness into the actual measurement process. Consciousness can affect micro- as well as macrocosmic phenomena according to quantum physicist Elizabeth Rauscher.[10] An expanded model of quantum physical processes involving conscious intervention was proposed by Dr. Rauscher. These include nonlinear processes in greater than four-dimensional space-time. Specifically, she describes a complex mathematical, eight-dimensional geometric space that contains a domain of action of local and nonlocal aspects of consciousness. This alternative theoretical approach might help us understand how the use of tuning forks in the biofield, as described in this book, could lead to the unique results that this author has been able to achieve, which on first examination seem to defy modern scientific and medical logic.

Sound transmission exists inside the body from the earliest moments of embryonic development inside the womb. These sonic symphonies and pulsations transmitted from the mother to the developing baby help shape its sense of hearing and develop the sense perceptions of vibration, touch, and texture. The latter senses form the major dorsal column pathways of the spine and the growing brain. Thus our whole nervous system is exquisitely conditioned from earliest development to absorb therapeutic modalities of vibration through acoustic and vibratory resonances. Indeed, when sound penetrates tissues, every molecule within the region of the body being treated shares in the sound data, including integral membrane proteins and even the DNA within the cells.[11] The environmental sound signals may act through epigenetic signaling processes yet to be defined to modulate the genome, the genetic code inside each cell nucleus, analogous to the other electromagnetic fields that can affect membrane proteins.[12]

Bioelectromagnetic researchers have found that digital electromagnetic pulses from our modern wireless devices can activate the voltage-gated calcium channels embedded in all cell membranes.[13] Today's plethora of modern microwave electromagnetic signals has been shown to have potentially adverse effects on our cells and tissues. The background microwave radiation in our environment from wireless communication technologies is especially high in our cities. Today this background radiation is nearly a million times higher than it was just thirty years ago before the advent of cell phones, cordless phones, WiFi, and wireless smart meters that are saturating the airwaves with microwave radiation. These technologies use pulsing electromagnetic fields that can adversely affect the nervous system and the brain. It is not unreasonable to suggest that pure analog sounds of continuous tones or melodious music might have the potential to correct the energetic imbalances that may be present in the body or the biofield of a person, perhaps even leading to the repair of imbalanced DNA or RNA genetic material in the cells.

This is an idea that is not at all purely speculative. In 2007 U.S. patent 7280874 was granted to Charlene Boehm for a method to determine therapeutic resonant frequencies in a variety of settings. These therapeutic resonant frequencies are claimed to be useful in modulating complete genomes and partial genomic materials and may be used in various media having different refractivities. If these ideas take hold in our modern medical system, there may come a time when sound healing will be as commonplace as modern pharmaceuticals are today. It is hoped that this book contributes in a significant way to a healing revolution using sound. May it find wide readership in North America and the rest of the world.

Dr. Karl H. Maret practices Complementary and Alternative Medicine (CAM), specializing in nutrition, functional medicine, and energy medicine. He holds an M.D. from the University of Toronto, a master's in biomedical engineering, and a bachelor of science in electrical engineering. He completed a four-year postdoctoral fellowship at the University of California, San Diego, and developed biomedical instrumentation for the successful 1981 American medical research expedition to Mt. Everest. Dr. Maret has lectured extensively in Europe and the United States on electromagnetic healing approaches, new water technologies, electrosmog challenges, and new integrative energy medicine therapies.

TRUTH HAS 144 SIDES

Biofield Tuning is a therapeutic method that makes use of the frequencies produced by tuning forks to detect and correct distortions and imbalances within the biomagnetic energy field, or biofield, that surrounds the human body. It is a process that has been evolving since I first picked up a set of tuning forks and began incorporating them into my massage therapy practice in 1996.

Biofield Tuning is based on the biofield anatomy hypothesis, the premise that our biofield, which extends approximately five feet on both sides of the body and three feet above the head and below the feet and is shaped like a torus, contains the record of all of our memories, embedded as energy and information in standing waves within this structure. Just as the brain is compartmentalized with different areas responsible for different functions, so is the biofield, with specific areas holding information related to specific emotions, states of mind, and relationships (see the Biofield Anatomy map in appendix C).

In addition to our memories, the biofield contains the blueprint that the physical body organizes itself around. Traumatic experiences on the physical, mental, and emotional levels give rise to pathological oscillations in the standing waves that act as a sort of noise in the signal and can cause a breakdown in the order, structure, and function of the physiology.

The tuning forks are used like sonar—as they are combed or passed through the field, their changing overtones reflect changes in the terrain of the biofield. Blockages of flow and distortions in the field show up as a dissonance that is readily perceived by both the therapist and the client. In this way they are used diagnostically. However, the coherent frequency of the forks also acts therapeutically in a very targeted way when the forks are held in specific areas of acute distortion, inducing greater order into the system.

In over twenty-five years of clinical practice, this method has shown itself to be beneficial for a wide range of symptoms: PTSD, anxiety, depression, pain, digestive disorders, vertigo, migraines, emotional discord, and more. It is gentle, noninvasive, simple, and efficient, and can be learned with relative ease. Its basic premise is that it assists the body and mind to relax out of habitual patterns of tension, imbalance, and stress response, and in doing so, facilitates self-healing.

While for the most part this process is subtle and gentle, it can also be surprisingly powerful. Readers should note from the outset that I have found a few situations where Biofield Tuning is contraindicated: when a pacemaker, pregnancy, or cancer is involved. It also does not appear appropriate for end-of-life or palliative care. Some sources cite metal screws, plates, and the like as contraindicated, but I have not found this to be a problem.

Sound can reset the rhythms of the body, which can interfere with the work of a pacemaker, so those with a pacemaker should consider avoiding this work. However, newer pacemakers are better shielded from outside influences and in some cases may not be a problem. Still, it is best to avoid working directly over any implanted electronics in the body to be on the safe side.

Pregnancy is contraindicated because of the detoxing potential of the work. While most people do not have strong detox reactions, some do, and this is something you do not want to put a pregnant woman through. Some weighted forks on the tight shoulders or sore feet of a mother-to-be are fine, but a full Biofield Tuning session of field combing, which I will describe later in this book, should be avoided.

This potential for detoxification is the same reason why those with cancer (or anyone who is very ill) should not undergo Biofield Tuning work. In truth, I have not done a whole lot of work with people who have cancer, but I have found that the work I have done with those who have it has left them exhausted. It's as if the body does not have the reserves to push the process through, and the energy just gets stuck. I would be willing to work with cancer patients in a facility where they are receiving other kinds of support, such as nutritional guidance, bodywork, and counseling, but Biofield Tuning as I have developed it does not work as a stand-alone practice for people who have a high degree of sickness, in my experience.

I have found that when I have shared these finding with my Biofield Tuning students, some become resistant to what I am saying and persist in wanting to work with people who have cancer and who are very sick. At the very least, if you have a loved one you want to help bring some relief to, keep in mind that in working with people with compromised systems, less is more. I do not suggest field combing in the area of the liver or kidneys or using the forks for more than fifteen or twenty minutes at a time. Think of it more in terms of helping them relax, rather than healing them.

People who are relatively healthy, however, often report more energy, greater clarity, a greater sense of equanimity, more inner peace, and the like. I have come to see that healing is a process of reclaiming our power and being able to experience greater degrees of freedom, and Biofield Tuning definitely supports this process.

But how does it? And why does it? What, exactly, is going on in a Biofield Tuning session? Does this pattern of the compartmentalized memory storage system that I have unwittingly uncovered in my research really exist? What laws of physics govern this structure and the way that sound interacts with it? What is the energy field composed of? These are questions I have been asking and seeking to understand ever since I first began using the forks, and especially in the last few years.

I have pursued this line of inquiry both independently and in more formal academic research for my master's thesis, which was titled "Exploring the Effects of Audible Sound on the Body and Its Biofield." Despite many years of hands-on clinical practice and many stacks of books that I have read, I still have more questions than answers and still consider myself more of a student than an expert in this field.

To that end, this book is more of a story, more art than science—the story of how and why I got into therapeutic sound, the development of a process I call Biofield Tuning, the story of my research and what I have learned, of how I discovered what I call the biofield anatomy (which you may find very valuable if you are a health or wellness provider), along with some client and student stories. It's the explanation of something that has arisen for the most part intuitively, the first stage in a process expressed nicely in this quote by scientist, statistician, and astrological researcher Michel Gauguelin: "The scientist knows that in the history of ideas, magic always precedes science, and the intuition of phenomena anticipates their objective knowledge."

It is my intention to apply the scientific method and some technological support to the process from here on, and to team with others who are asking the same sorts of questions, so that my subsequent efforts in this field should provide us with more answers (and no doubt, more questions). But in the meantime, before we get to that place where science will reveal to us a more objective understanding of what I will share here, we are faced with skepticism of the unknown.

SCIENCE AND SPIRIT

As I am writing this, TED Talks (Technology, Entertainment, Design), a popular televised forum for "spreading ideas worth sharing," counsels us to avoid anything that seeks to unify science and spirituality. In seeking to understand the science of the subtle energy field that appears to surround the body, I am potentially doing exactly what they are advising against. What is the peculiar cultural aversion to this unification?

I recently asked my son's teenage friend to say the first thing that came to mind when I said "energy medicine," and his reply was "taboo." This division of metaphysical and physical, of woo-woo and not woo-woo, in some ways defines our culture: there are those in the metaphysical camp and those in the scientific camp. What would it mean for this division to dissolve?

Perhaps because I was born under the sign of Libra, a sign characterized by its desire to seek to balance and harmonize opposites, I have been troubled by the divide between science and spirit ever since I was a teenager. And, as such, I have sought to both understand the divide and do what I can to reconcile it—a territory that, according to the folks at TED, apparently is verboten, and anyone reporting from this territory is suspect and not to be trusted. I didn't understand why the divide has held so fast until while doing research for my thesis I came across a passage in a scholarly article that stated that the English translations of words chi, qi, prana, and the like, terms found in other languages to designate subtle energy, include "spirit" and "Holy Spirit." Since modern science is forbidden to go there—spirit is purportedly the domain of religion, not science—the dividing line falls squarely at the boundary of what we call energy or subtle energy.

Here are some of the reasons for this dividing line, as outlined by Scott Virdin Anderson, M.D., in his article "The Emerging Science of Subtle Energy":

- There is *no agreed-upon scientific definition* of subtle energy, and hence *no reliable methodology* for detecting or measuring the energies so defined.
- There is *no broadly accepted scientific theory* of such energies.
- The very notion of subtle energy *originates in prescientific esoteric traditions,* which have been systematically marginalized by scientific enterprises for more than a century.
- The notion is thus considered far *too subjective,* or worse, *a point of religious belief,* or worse yet, *a mere superstition.*[1]

The resolution of this conundrum is fairly simple—all we need is a scientific definition of subtle energy, and, bingo, no more divide! However, there are many powerful forces that have vested interests in maintaining the status quo, making what should be simple fairly complicated. One of these is the skeptic.

THE VALUE OF SKEPTICISM

Dr. Gary Schwartz, professor of psychology, medicine, neurology, psychiatry, and surgery at the University of Arizona and director of its Laboratory for Advances in Consciousness and Health, distinguishes between what he calls "true skeptics" and "pseudo-skeptics":

> True skeptics not only know that they don't know something for sure, but they are genuinely open to changing their minds and growing in light of new evidence. In a deep sense they are humble and open-minded. Pseudo-skeptics often are typically disbelievers—i.e., they are firmly entrenched in believing "no" about certain things. Although they may "claim" that they are open to new information, they typically react with strongly unfriendly if not hostile criticisms when their beliefs and assumptions are challenged by new ideas and evidence.[2]

We all have the skeptic in us to different degrees. It has been put there by our education, by advertising, by the flavor of our culture. I have it in me. I am actually very skeptical by nature and always have been. I remember my mother exclaiming regularly, with exasperation, "You can't tell that child anything, she has to figure it out for herself!" It's true—I don't like to take other people's words for things. I like to investigate a subject thoroughly, determine what makes sense, what rings true, and form my own perspective on it. Even then I am always open to new ideas that might make more sense.

In science, truth is, ideally, an evolving process, not an absolute destination. Yet truth be told, even after twenty-five years of using tuning forks, I still sometimes cringe when I see other people using them.

The thing is, if my work with forks hadn't been so fascinating, hadn't produced such compelling results, I never would have stuck with it all these years.

I have witnessed many extraordinary and powerful shifts in people from this work: the diminishment or eradication of pain, anxiety, digestive distress, vertigo, restless-leg syndrome, panic attacks, and various forms of "stuckness." Headaches, TMJ, back tension, knee issues, and herpes outbreaks have all been lessened or dissipated totally through Biofield Tuning. The work I have done with people suffering from PTSD and symptoms from concussions has been particularly compelling. I have found that this is an efficient, elegant, noninvasive process, and an interesting means of demonstrating that there does indeed appear to be a field of energy and information that surrounds the body.

The fact of the matter is that when it comes to subtle energy, the person who considers him- or herself to be a skeptic often isn't really a true skeptic. Rather, he or she is simply reacting from what they've been told, being what Dr. Schwartz refers to as a "pseudo-skeptic." On occasion I have asked some of these folks, "Have you determined that the scientific method has shown concretely that subtle energy does not exist? Have you read studies that have shown that audible sound has no discernible therapeutic effect on the body? Why are you so certain that your knee-jerk response is valid—because other people have told you this and you believe them? Where is your skepticism about what you have been told?"

What we have all been told goes something like this:

Human bodies do not have an energy field, in fact, there's not even any such thing as an energy field. Fields are constructs in which some direction or intensity is measured at every point: gravity, wind, magnetism, some expression of energy. Energy is just a measurement; it doesn't exist on its own as a cloud or a field or some other entity. The notion that frequencies can interact with the body's energy field is, as the saying goes, so wrong it's not even wrong.[3]

These kinds of statements, delivered as facts, directly contradict what my senses explicitly tell me. Not just mine, but those of pretty much everyone who has ever received a session or a lesson from me. Yet we are often told that we cannot believe our own senses, that they are not to be trusted. Instead we must listen to the "experts" (i.e., the scientists who tell us what is and what is not valid). It's amazing to me how many people do not trust their own senses, and yet—here's another paradox—skeptics will often not believe something until they hear it with their own ears, see it with their own eyes, and in fact perceive it with their own senses. Then they believe.

We also are confronted with the issue of semantics. In fact, I would go so far as to say that words are our biggest problem here. There is a lot of confusion and even hostility from the skeptic around words like energy, frequency, quantum, and such. So we have to define and agree on the definitions of some terms before we start throwing them around. To this end, I recently came across this quote by Paul John Rosch, chairman of the board of the American Institute of Stress, clinical professor of medicine and psychiatry at New York Medical College, and honorary vice president of the International Stress Management Association:

> There is an unfortunate tendency to believe that just because you have given something a name, that somehow you have defined it—or worse, that everyone will understand what it means. *Stress* is a good example; after almost fifty years in the field, I can assure you that attempting to define or explain stress to a scientist's satisfaction is like trying to nail a piece of jelly to a tree. Hans Selye, who coined the term *stress* as it is currently used and struggled with this problem his entire life, was fond of pointing out that "everyone knows what stress is, but nobody really knows."[4]

The best way to know about anything is by examining it from multiple perspectives. Like the analogy of the blind men examining the elephant (see figure I.1), it takes many visions married together to see the big picture.

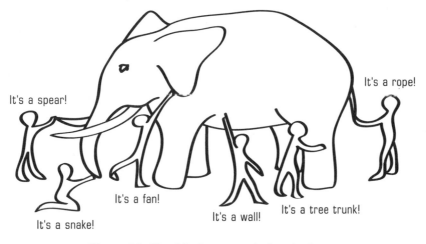

Figure I.1. The blind men and the elephant
Illustration by Kimberly Lipinski

THE MANY FACETS OF TRUTH

At one point in conducting research, I came across the concept of biophotons and became quite interested in them, reading everything I could find on the subject and also watching some YouTube videos. One of the videos I came across was of Dr. Johan Boswinkel of the Netherlands talking about biophoton therapy, a method he had developed. This learned man had so many profound things to say in the first ten minutes of this lecture that I actually had to stop it to go get a notebook and then restart it so I could take notes.

Among his many pearls of wisdom, Dr. Boswinkel said, without much elaboration, "I believe that truth has 144 sides."

That enigmatic statement stuck in my brain like an arrow. I could not stop thinking about it for days. Truth has 144 sides? What does that mean? The more I thought about it, the more it began to profoundly shape my outlook. If this is so, then what I perceive is just a facet, a sliver of the "truth" of any given situation. Suddenly, other people's perspectives, rather than being something to argue against, seemed crucial to my understanding of things. I stopped arguing with my husband (well, mostly, anyway), because

I suddenly had much greater appreciation for his perspective than I had previously had.

It also made me think of the so-called Dunbar's number of roughly 150, named after British anthropologist Robin Dunbar. This refers to the cognitive limit to the number of people with whom one can maintain stable social relationships, meaning relationships in which each person knows who every other person is and how each person relates to every other person. It has been observed that numbers larger than this generally require more restrictive rules to maintain a stable, cohesive group.

Dunbar's observations of various villages, tribes, and groups included the estimated sizes of a Neolithic farming village, the splitting point of Hutterite (a group similar to the Amish) settlements, the basic unit size of the Roman army, and approximations of the ideal size of a company or company division. Numerous studies point to the legitimacy of his theory. So this concept of ideal size of a human community or organization and the concept of truth being a construct that has 144 sides makes me think that we need the individual perspectives of that many people to form a cohesive framework of collective functioning. Every person's perspective is necessary and valid, but obviously different.

MY PERSPECTIVE

I offer this concept as an olive branch of sorts, because my experience has revealed to me a way of perceiving that is contrary to both conventional beliefs about the nature of mind and the biofield, as well as the esoteric view. In a nutshell, I have come to believe that the memories of our life experience are recorded not in the brain, but rather in a sort of magnetic fashion in the bioplasmic bubble of our biofield (i.e., the human energy field, or aura), and that this field is compartmentalized and follows a timeline (as we generate information it moves away from our center toward our periphery, like rings in a tree). I'll go into this in much more detail in subsequent chapters.

In the course of trying to understand the phenomena that I have encountered working around the body with tuning forks, I have uncovered an entirely different cosmology, the big picture about the nature of life. It includes the abandoned concept of aether and the surprisingly ignored concept of plasma, and needless to say it goes against our conventional model. Because this perspective is unusual and doesn't fit into our current scientific and materialist paradigm, we have to spend time looking at and redefining the paradigm so that it does fit. We end up having to contemplate a lot more than just audible sound and how and why it can be applied therapeutically to the human body.

What are the credentials I have that inform my perspective? As a child I was considered gifted and was moved ahead a few grades so that I graduated from high school when I was sixteen. At that age I had no idea what I wanted to study and so refrained from going to college, instead choosing to work and save money to travel, then to begin and then sell a few different successful businesses, then start a family, until it finally occurred to me, at age thirty-seven, that I wanted to be a teacher at the college level, and to do that I needed a few degrees. So in 2007 I entered college as an adult learner. I had the good fortune to participate in a program called Assessment of Prior Learning (APL) that is taught through Community College of Vermont (CCV). APL offers college credit for thoroughly documented life experiences. Through this program and a few other classes at CCV, I received enough credits to enter Northern Vermont University here in my hometown in Vermont, as a senior.

Because of my diverse background in both business and healing, the degree I ended up with is in general studies, although my electives were in the Wellness and Alternative Medicine program, one of the few such programs in a public undergraduate college in the country. I must confess to a bit of embarrassment around the title of my undergraduate degree (they have since changed the name to Professional Studies). We live in a culture that applauds and rewards specialists, and so to be a generalist—which I very much am—is not so highly esteemed. My master's degree, also from Northern Vermont University, is in education, and since I pursued an independent, nonlicensure track, I was able to customize it to my own interests somewhat. I called my independent track "Integrative Education" and pursued independent studies, looking at that which connects the disciplines. An integrative viewpoint looks at how things connect to one another, instead of the traditional academic route that tends to yield specialists, not generalists.

So, academically I am credentialed to teach things of a general nature relating to health and wellness and the interrelatedness of things, which is largely what I am doing in this book. I am, however, also a specialist of sorts from my many years of independent research, specifically on how therapeutically applied pure acoustic frequencies affect the body and mind. I will go into this in some detail in this book.

Not to argue for my limitations, but it seems to be a general trend that when you are gifted in one area you often suffer a detriment in others. I love words and books and learning, but I am completely hopeless when it comes to math. The parts of the brain that help you to understand higher math concepts—music, chess, anything requiring spatial intelligence—these parts are nearly inaccessible to me. I remember a particularly traumatic event in fifth grade, of not being able to comprehend long division to save my life, which was the first time I was confronted with my dyslexia. I spent many frustrating months struggling to make my way through division worksheets, suffering quite a blow to my ego, since I had been accustomed up to this point to being a "child genius," out in front of everyone on the learning curve of almost any subject. I don't transpose words or letters like the more common form of dyslexia; I transpose numbers, left and right, random things like *Star Wars* and *Star Trek,* and even the names of my son's friends Henry and Andy.

So in my quest to better understand life, the universe, and what it means to be a human being, especially a healthy human being, all subjects of interest to me since I was a teenager, I have had to bypass the math route simply because it boggles my mind and I can't seem to get beyond it, despite trying very hard. Because of this I skipped physics and chemistry and every math class I could possibly avoid in high school and college. Given that math and science are very much in favor at the moment as the means of investigating these sorts of things, I have had to seek to understand and communicate my understanding of these things in words.

To that end, I have done quite a lot of reading—I would say that I have pretty much had a nonfiction book or three on my bedside table since I was eighteen years old, for the last thirty-four years. Recently, my son Quinn came into my room with a novel that he had just finished, suggesting I read it. I nodded toward my usual pile of research books and told him I had plenty to read at the moment. "Mom," he said, "even Vulcans read literature." I agreed that he had a point and tried to start the novel, but my brain was back to asking questions about things, and before I knew it my nose was back in nonfiction.

So, my perspective is informed by a lot of reading, especially what, for lack of a better term, has been called New Age science, which has been particularly interesting to me. The division between science and religion, between the secular and spiritual, is an invisible yet powerful divider that separates us. It's a curious construct, like gang turf. People tend to gravitate to one side or the other. But does anyone really know what the other side is talking about? Words like *energy* and *quantum* and *God* and *soul* are thrown about, and lots of people get emotional, but really, what the heck are we talking about? Maybe we're talking about the same thing but using different words. Maybe there really is only one truth and we all need to hear one another in order to see it.

It's not about the words, anyway; it's about the underlying vibrational patterning, the tone, the subjective inner electromagnetic experience that is your perception, which we seek to understand and describe with words. We've all gotten so lost in the words that we have forgotten that they are a poor approximation for deeper truths. So on that note, in chapter 1, we'll be taking a look at some of the words we will be using in this practice.

1

THE POWER OF WORDS

Redefining Our Assumptions by Returning to the Basics

Any problem, big or small, always seems to start with bad communication. Someone isn't listening.

EMMA THOMPSON

The therapeutic use of sound falls into a category called *energy medicine*. It could also be called *sound medicine, vibrational medicine, sound healing, sound therapy, frequency medicine, integrative medicine, alternative medicine,* and probably other names besides. That alone is confusing. Let's start with the term *energy medicine* and break it down into its components.

Here is the *Webster's Dictionary* definition of the word *energy:*

1. The capacity for vigorous activity; available power
2. A feeling of having an adequate or abundant amount of such power
3. An exertion of such power; effort: *threw her energies into the job*
4. The habit of vigorous activity; vigor
5. The ability to act, lead others, or effect things forcefully
6. Forcefulness of expression
7. *Physics:* the capacity to do work; symbol: E
8. A source of usable power, as fossil fuel or electricity

None of these definitions really explain the energy we are talking about in energy medicine. So that is part of the problem—there is, as we said earlier, no real standardized definition of the term as it is used here. These are all definitions from our scientific and materialist paradigm, and within this paradigm the energy in *energy medicine* is, well, undefined. So, for our purposes in moving forward, we need to give it a definition. This is a surprisingly complicated endeavor, and no doubt this complication is why we have yet to collectively do so in a way that everyone seems to agree on.

WHAT IS ENERGY?

Pure energy is electromagnetic radiation, light. It is simply frequency, movement—or put another way, *sound*. (We'll get to the definition of this word in a bit.) Ultimately, everything comes from the stars, which are made of *plasma* (and we'll define this word later too). And ultimately, everything can return to its plasma state by being burned. So everything is really just some form of embodied light when you get right down to it.

Look around you. Everything you see is energy. This book, the chair in which you are sitting, the building you are in, the planet you are on, the solar system, the universe—it is all ultimately electromagnetic energy vibrating at different frequencies. Every single thing in our observable universe is in motion, even things apparently not moving, like rocks. We all know that at an atomic and subatomic level, the rock is in constant motion. In the words of the late, great physicist Richard Feynman, "Everything jiggles." We could just as easily say, "Everything jitterbugs," which would actually be a more appropriate definition because it is the dynamic interplay between the positive and negative forces that gives rise to this dance of energy.

Even though energy is technically broken down into different categories—thermal, chemical, kinetic, potential, and others—for the purposes of this conversation when we refer to *energy* we are speaking of electromagnetic energy. But what of subtle energy? What exactly is subtle energy? This is also a difficult subject, one that many people have tried to define, again leading to a whole lot of different words and no simple, clear definition.

Here are some of the words that people use to define these subtle energies: *chi, ki, prana, orgone, od, tachyon, aether, Akasha, longitudinal waves, Tesla waves, scalar waves, spirit, Holy Spirit, zero-point field, the implicate order, the Higgs field, the source field, the torsion field, the field, gravity waves, neutrinos.* Again, confusing!

The way I have come to see it is that subtle energy is the same as electromagnetism in that it is just light, but different in that it is light at very high (and possibly very low) frequencies, where it behaves differently and responds to different laws. For example, people who have done studies on subtle energy have observed that like attracts like, meaning positive charges are attracted to other positive charges and vice versa, but at a certain key threshold of frequency this flips, and then opposites attract.

One analogy that comes to mind is that subtle energy is to our current understanding of electricity, also referred to as classical electromagnetism, as water vapor or steam is to water; it is essentially the same thing, only finer, more diffuse, and it obeys different laws. At a certain key threshold the form of water changes: 32 degrees Fahrenheit to freeze, 212 degrees to turn to steam. Subtle energy is present everywhere electromagnetic energy is present, just as water vapor is present wherever water is. And just as water vapor is diffuse water, subtle energy is diffuse electromagnetism. You can't measure subtle energy with a volt meter any more than you can measure water vapor with a measuring cup.

Another perspective, one that is a little harder to grasp, is that this energy propagates differently than classical electromagnetism, moving in longitudinal rather than transverse waves. Transverse waves propagate or travel up and down at 90-degree angles to the direction they are traveling (see figure 1.1). Longitudinal waves propagate in the direction they are going without going up and down. Sound is described as a

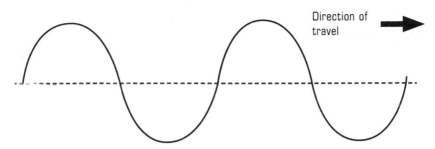

Figure 1.1. Transverse wave

Figure 1.2. Longitudinal wave

longitudinal wave but is generally depicted as a transverse sine wave (see figure 1.2).

Generally, electromagnetism is seen as a transverse wave and not assigned any longitudinal properties. James Clerk Maxwell (1831–1879) was a Scottish theoretical physicist whose theories and mathematic equations demonstrated that electricity, magnetism, and light are all manifestations of the same phenomenon: the electromagnetic field. What is lesser known about Maxwell's work is that in his original twenty equations, he had formulas for these longitudinal waves as well. However, the equations were rewritten and simplified to just four by British mathematician and physicist Oliver Heaviside (1850–1925). These four equations are what we use today, and they do not include the equations for the longitudinal aspects that Maxwell perceived and sought to describe.

It would appear that subtle energy may simply be a currently unrecognized form of electromagnetism, as the formulas that describe it have been erased from contemporary science. It is these frequencies that may comprise what we know as *subtle energy.*

Let's take another look at a few of the different words listed earlier and learn a bit about them.

Chi and *ki* are respectively the Chinese and Japanese words that most simply are defined as "the life force inherent in all things." This life force is seen as both circulating through the body and the Earth in yin (feminine/negative) and yang (masculine/positive) forms. *Prana* is the Sanskrit word for the same concept, and *ka* is the ancient Egyptian word for it. *Orgone* was the name given to it by Austrian psychoanalyst Wilhelm Reich, and *od* was the name assigned by German chemist, geologist, and metallurgist Carl Von Reichenbach. *Aether* is the classical term for it, as in the *luminiferous aether* (or *ether*), the liquid light medium that fills all of space. The concept of aether was largely a given in science until it was excised in the early part of the last century.

Ultimately, what each of these words describes is the same phenomenon: high-frequency energies (and perhaps very low frequencies as well) that are present everywhere all at once, can be present in different densities and charges, behave in ways that have been successfully studied and replicated by scientists all over the world, and are the ultimate ground state from which all explicate or visible phenomena arise. Another property ascribed to subtle energy in many of these definitions is consciousness. Here is another one of our slippery words. We'll define *consciousness* in a moment, but first let's finish with *energy.*

So, for the purpose of this book, when I refer to energy in the context of energy medicine, I am referring to both classical electromagnetism (as described by the four Heaviside equations) as well as subtle energy. I'll use a few of the other terms to allude to subtle energy as well—*chi, aether,* and *life force.* While our current popular science claims that these energies do not exist—the biggest reason being they have not been measured—we are going to suspend this disbelief for several reasons: If millions or perhaps billions of people throughout time and around the world have perceived and described these energies, and there is a common denominator in all of these descriptions, there must be some validity to it. We have been acculturated to believe that our current scientific perspective is the pinnacle of thought and evolution, and that if current science says that there is no life force, no energy fields, then this must be true. And it may be true. However, when one takes a really good look at the evidence, especially the evidence we find "under the rug," that subtle energy does indeed exist is fairly hard to deny. The biggest reason it continues to be denied by the academy (i.e., our educational system), from what I can tell, is that it has a history of being denied. Western education is rooted in the separation of science and spirit, which means that solids, liquids, and gases are "real," and the higher and finer frequencies that one might call *soul* or *spirit* are "not real."

This view is especially prevalent when it comes to our prevailing system of medicine. Medical science, in particular, largely looks at life in terms of solids, liquids, and gases alone. Which brings us to the word *medicine* . . .

WHAT IS MEDICINE?

Here's the definition from *Webster's:*

1. The science of diagnosing, treating, or preventing disease and other damage to the body or mind; the branch of this science encompassing treatment by drugs, diet, exercise, and other non-surgical means
2. The practice of medicine
3. An agent, such as a drug, used to treat disease or injury
4. Something that serves as a remedy or corrective: *medicine for rebuilding the economy; measures that were harsh medicine*
5. Shamanistic practices or beliefs, especially among Native Americans; something, such as a ritual practice or sacred object,

believed to control natural or supernatural powers or serve as a
preventive or remedy

This is a good broad definition that includes shamanic practices
and beliefs; shamans are the original sound healers, who, with song
and chant and drum and rattle and didgeridoo, harness the power of
sound in healing. While sound can be purely physical in its benefits,
like relieving pain or improving digestion, it can also be healing on
what we might call a spiritual level. It works with both classic and
subtle energy.

So anything that helps bring about healing, or a shift from an
incoherent, unhealthy state to a coherent, healthy state, can be called
medicine. Our current model of allopathic medicine—drugs and
surgery—treats the body as a machine and eliminates from the equation the consciousness that animates the body. Which brings us back
to consciousness.

WHAT IS CONSCIOUSNESS?

Let's see what *Webster's* has to say about consciousness:

1. The state of being conscious; awareness
2. The thoughts and feelings, collectively, of an individual or of an
   aggregate of people
3. Full activity of the mind and senses, as in waking life: *to regain
   consciousness*
4. Awareness of something for what it is; internal knowledge:
   consciousness of wrongdoing
5. Concern, interest, or awareness: *class consciousness*
6. The mental activity of which a person is aware, contrasted with
   unconscious thought
7. *Philosophy:* the mind or the mental faculties, characterized by
   thought, feelings, and volition

Essentially, the paradigm or worldview that we, in our Western culture, are educated into (called *scientific materialism*) teaches us that consciousness arises from the activity in the brain, is completely local to and within our bodies, and dissolves at death along with the physical body. We have no eternal soul, there is no heaven and hell, and there is no God. An alternative perspective on this is that consciousness precedes the human body, survives after death, and that the body exists within our consciousness. The question is, is consciousness the function of what we would call our *soul* (another slippery word) or what we call our *brain?* How can we really know?

When it comes right down to it, right here and now, we don't really know, inasmuch as there is no scientific consensus on the subject beyond the assumption that consciousness arises in the brain, so any science that shows otherwise is unlikely to make it into peer-reviewed journals. I want to make it clear that I am referring to mainstream science, or popular science from a layman's perspective. I am aware that there are many people in academia who are taking a good, hard look at this right now, but it has yet to trickle down into our popular perception.

"We know people have ideas beyond the mainstream," said the sociologist Harriet Zuckerman, author of *Scientific Elite: Nobel Laureates in the United States* and senior vice president of the Andrew W. Mellon Foundation, "but if they want funds for research they have to go through peer review, and the system is going to be very skeptical of ideas that are inconsistent with what is already known."[1]

As you can see from this quote, the research funding and peer-review process is largely set up to reinforce its own assumptions. One of the talks that *TED* removed from their TEDx YouTube channel (and then reinstated after public outcry) was given by British scientist, prolific author, and researcher Rupert Sheldrake, who summarized the ideas he presented his book *Science Set Free,* in which he questions what he calls the "ten dogmas, or assumptions, of scientific materialism." One of these assumptions is that other than human beings, nothing else has consciousness. It should be noted, however, that last year a group of prominent scientists got together and agreed that animals do have consciousness, so at least we are getting somewhere! However, science has yet to ascribe sentience to trees, rocks, water, or stars: all of these things are not conscious. This goes against the beliefs of indigenous peoples everywhere, who have lived in much greater harmony with the natural world before the corrupting influence of the white man appeared.

The bottom line is that we can't look to current reductionist science to tell us anything about consciousness beyond the fact that it supposedly originates in the brain and dies when our bodies die. There is a steadfast unwillingness to look beyond this assumption because this would mean looking at spirit or subtle energy, and science is forbidden to go there: that territory falls into the category of spirituality. This separation of science and spirit has been going on for hundreds of years and in some ways has been useful, but it also has its limitations.

This is what Sheldrake is calling out and getting persecuted for. He's saying let's look at these assumptions and how they get in the way of science really moving forward, instead of stubbornly defending them as some sort of doctrine. Let's take a scientific look at subtle energy instead of just dismissing it as not existing. There's plenty of evidence—mountains, actually—that human intention can influence random number generators, that energy healing produces consistently beneficial outcomes in lab mice, that ordinary people can sense when they are being stared at, that distant viewing can be highly accurate. And if we look to other traditions, we see ample evidence that supports the theory of the eternal soul that carries on, reanimating different bodies in its journey through time. As of this writing, there is a very popular book written by neurosurgeon Eben Alexander titled *Proof of Heaven: A Neurosurgeon's Journey into the Afterlife,* which is currently a number-one bestseller. Alexander was a successful scientific reductionist who was of the belief that consciousness arose in the brain until he had a profound near-death experience that showed him otherwise. And while ultimately a book such as this can't really offer tangible proof, its popularity speaks volumes about people's hunger to hear that they really do have eternal souls.

The fact of the matter is that we can't really know what happens after death, whether there is such a thing as heaven or hell, if you reincarnate or simply dissolve back into the cosmic soup with your atoms reincarnating as part of a worm and some dirt and a tree. I've been on the fence about reincarnation for most of my practice because, as a practical skeptic, I don't generally form beliefs about things I cannot see clear evidence of. This is in contrast to my opinion about subtle energy because I have had my hands in it for years and my experience correlates with the reported experiences of countless others.

Because consciousness is described as being a property of subtle energy, and science denies the existence of subtle energy, it's easy to see why it's such a slippery widget to describe and understand. Sometimes when I am stumped in my understanding of things, I ask my children. I have gotten lots of insights from engaging my boys in my philosophical wonderings, and so while writing about this, I asked my kids, who both had friends over, what they thought the word *consciousness* meant. The youngest one in the house, my son's friend who is ten, immediately quipped, "being aware of your needs or wants." My twelve-year-old said "self-awareness." The older two confused what I was asking with the word *conscience:* "Oh, you know, the part of you that tells you to do the right thing even though you might be willfully doing the wrong thing."

This perspective leads me to this quote by Thoreau: "I believe there is a subtle magnetism in nature, which if we unconsciously yield to it, will guide us aright." Looked at from this perspective, our conscience is a gentle nudge seeking to guide us into alignment with the larger consciousness that is present everywhere.

Try a little experiment: Imagine that you have a luminous, expansive aspect to yourself that we'll call *consciousness* and that it cannot die and furthermore that it is connected luminously to all that is. Now imagine that you don't—that you are a tiny individual unit in a meaningless, disconnected world, and once it's over, it's over. Which scenario feels better?

Now imagine that you own a very powerful business selling pills to help people who feel depressed, powerless, and scared, and that you fund research that helps to shape the collective perception of reality. From a business perspective, which worldview would you want your research to cultivate? We have to be realistic when we look at funded research and the peer-review process and what it comes up with, because while there are genuinely curious people seeking knowledge for knowledge's sake, there is also a very significant component of research driven by corporate interests seeking to create profits.

There is a statement from Karl Marx that "religion is the opiate of the masses." In this case, choosing to align oneself with the spiritual belief that we have an immortal soul that gets to keep trying on a human suit until we master the experience is comforting. It feels, for many people, a lot better than the alternative. It could be said to be an opiate of sorts, one that if you are very aligned with it, regardless of the belief system in which it is framed, creates a sort of bliss that eschews the need for antidepressants.

So, coming back to the definition of the word *consciousness,* again for the purpose of our discussion here, we are going to assume that consciousness is self-awareness, and that all living things experience it to some degree, and that even things we consider inorganic possess a degree of it as well. It implies an additional dimension beyond our little "meat machine," where we have the potential to connect to the greater consciousness, or all that is. Whether it continues on after death and in what way remains open to debate.

How we choose to frame our experience of consciousness is largely dependent on our paradigm. So now, let's look at the word *paradigm.*

WHAT IS A PARADIGM?

Here's *Webster's* again: "A philosophical and theoretical framework of a scientific school or discipline within which theories, laws, and generalizations and the experiments performed in support of them are formulated; broadly, a philosophical or theoretical framework of any kind."

Here's another definition: "A paradigm is a worldview, a general perspective, a way of breaking down the complexity of the real world. As such, paradigms are deeply imbedded in the socialization of adherents and practitioners: paradigms tell them what is important, legitimate, and reasonable."[2]

Currently we are educated into the framework of scientific materialism, which looks at life in terms of solids, liquids, and gases; sees the universe and everything in it as a machine; denies the existence of subtle energy and all of the phenomena associated with it (such as remote viewing, remote healing, telepathy, synchronicity, and the like); and generally sees everything as being separate and separated, including one's mind and one's body.

The concepts of the soul, spirit, subtle energy, unity consciousness, and even, as I have found, Biofield Tuning, don't fit into our conventional paradigm. Again, we find people dividing into camps on this subject. Most people accept what they are told without questioning it or looking beyond it. But for those of us who stubbornly insist on questioning what we are told, there is something dissatisfyingly incomplete and even depressing about our official paradigm.

It was this sense that I wasn't being told the whole story, and that not knowing the whole story was contributing to me not being healthy, that has been the driver in my quest to see the big picture and that has led me, somewhat unexpectedly, to the next level, if you will, beyond paradigm: to cosmology.

WHAT IS COSMOLOGY?

Webster's says:

1. A branch of metaphysics that deals with the nature of the universe; a theory or doctrine describing the natural order of the universe

2. A branch of astronomy that deals with the origin, structure, and space-time relationships of the universe; also, a theory dealing with these matters

I would add another definition: the study of the universe in its totality and by extension, human beings' role in it. Interestingly, cosmology is a subject we don't hear much about, particularly in school. Our assumptions about the nature of reality and the universe inform all of the sciences—each and every human discipline is influenced by our governing cosmology. It sets the stage on which the human drama is played out.

Our understanding of the universe and our relationship to it gives rise to our values, which define and guide the choices we make. It's because of this that it's an important concept to examine, and yet it goes largely unexamined; in our culture, in our age of specialists, the philosophical cosmologist is largely unheard of. I'm going to talk a lot about cosmology as we go on because in all of my research and studies, I have found that it is a field that I resonate with most strongly, and so I find it is important that we take a really good look at it.

A few years ago, when I was driving my then-thirteen-year-old son to school, he asked me, "Mom, are you a sound healer or a physicist?"

I replied, "Well, I am a sound healer who is trying to understand the physics of sound healing. But really what I am is a cosmological storyteller."

"I think I'll just tell people you're a physicist," he said.

It's easy to see why my son would prefer to tell his friends and teachers that his mother is a physicist. A scientist is a valid and esteemed member of our community, physicists especially so. A sound healer, like the term *energy medicine,* immediately raises a red flag. I know this firsthand. When I first committed to choosing therapeutic sound as my primary vocation and I told people that I was a sound healer, I almost always perceived a subtle but perceptible ideological rejection by most people. Even when I changed it to *sound therapist,* there was a kind of skeptical dismissal, an I've-never-heard-of-that dismissal. I finally got smart and changed it to *researcher who has been studying the effects of audible sound on the human body*. This is very well received by everyone. "Oh, you're a scientist (I approve). What have you learned?" It wouldn't make sense to tell people that I am a cosmological storyteller because nobody would know what that means—and it sounds sort of silly, so I keep that to myself. But of all the different hats I have worn and facets I have (my husband calls me "the woman of 10,000 epitaphs"), it is what resonates most deeply with me.

What I have learned from the great pile of books I have read and the many teachers I have learned from, and the direct insights from synthesizing all of this information, goes far beyond simply understanding the hows and whys of therapeutic sound. It is that our prevailing cosmological story is not only wrong and limited and largely unexamined, but also subconsciously destructive, depressing, and disempowering, and that when people learn of this new cosmology, they become very excited and energized.

I recently gave some lectures in New York City called "Electric You, Electric Universe," in which I introduced this new cosmology. (To give you a sense of just how much more I have become interested in philosophical cosmology as opposed to sound, the PowerPoint presentation of this lecture has sixty-two slides about cosmology and three on how it relates to Biofield Tuning.) Telling the story of this new cosmology to people is such an interesting process. "This is the missing piece," people told me. "This is so exciting and inspiring!" It makes many things fall into place for people, and the number-one thing I have heard each time I give this lecture is, "This makes sense."

Our cosmology should make sense. It should resonate with us on a deep level. When we hear it, we should know that we know it, even though we may not have learned it yet. It shouldn't be hard to understand.

And this brings me to my next word, which I have found very hard to understand: *quantum*.

QUANTUM, AN OVERUSED WORD?

One of the classic skeptic gripes I have come across is the way that alternative proponents use the word *quantum* in their description of methods and materials relating to alternative practices. I have chosen to not use this word much, if at all, in my practice and in this book, and there are several reasons why.

One is that despite many attempts at forays into quantum physics, I still don't really get what it is saying, other than the quotes I have cherry-picked that support my "everything is ultimately frequencies" perspective. I bought my son a book called *Alice in Quantum Land* in the hopes that we would both read it and together emerge with an understanding of quantum physics. Maybe this is one of the places where my dyslexia kicks in, but every time I try to go there, I feel like I am traversing a swamp.

Let's look at *Webster's* definition of the word *quantum:*

1. Quantity, amount; portion, part; gross quantity; bulk
2. Any of the very small increments or parcels into which many forms of energy are subdivided; any of the small subdivisions of a quantized physical magnitude (as magnetic moment)

So basically *quantum* means the tiniest of the tiny. Okay, then quantum physics: "the study of physics at the subatomic scale." But that doesn't really tell us much, does it?

Here is an interesting definition from "A Lazy Layman's Guide to Quantum Physics." The writer, James Higgo, a critical thinker and renaissance man who philosophized about life, including quantum physics, says that the following statements can be derived from the findings of quantum physics:

Your consciousness affects the behavior of subatomic particles

—or—

Particles move backwards as well as forwards in time and appear in all possible places at once

—or—

The universe is splitting, every Planck-time (10 E-43 seconds) into billions of parallel universes

—or—

The universe is interconnected with faster-than-light transfers of information.[3]

Higgo goes on to explain that the trouble with quantum physics—why it feels like a swamp to a casual observer like myself—is that there are many different interpretations of what it is. I could go on in detail to describe some of the different interpretations, but that would be wading into exactly the kind of confusing complexity we are hoping to avoid. If you would like to know more about quantum physics, feel free to investigate it and form your own opinion. I, for one, am going to choose to mostly avoid bringing it into this discussion.

However, before I came to this conclusion, to illustrate my point as to why sound is a useful therapeutic medium, I have used the following quote by quantum physicist Max Planck, who, upon receiving the Nobel Prize for physics in 1918, said, "We have now discovered that there is no such thing as matter; it is all just different rates of vibration designed by an unseen intelligence." It is quotes such as this, which I consider pop quantum physics, that informed my sense that since everything is ultimately vibration, including the human body, then treating vibration with vibration is logical and elegant.

Another word for *vibration* is *frequency*. Let's take a look at this one.

WHAT IS A FREQUENCY?

Here's the definition from *Merriam-Webster's:*

The number of waves that pass a fixed point per unit time; also, the number of cycles or vibrations undergone in unit time by a body in periodic motion. Frequency f is the reciprocal of the time T taken to complete one cycle (the period), or $1/T$. The frequency with which Earth rotates is once per 24 hours. Frequency is usually expressed in units called hertz (Hz). One hertz is equal to one cycle per second; one kilohertz (kHz) is 1,000 Hz, and one megahertz (MHz) is 1,000,000 Hz.

So frequency is simply the amount of vibrations within a particular amount of time. I have a variety of frequencies of tuning forks, for example. Since everything jiggles, or jitterbugs, everything, therefore, has a frequency. Each organ and each system in our body resonates at a particular frequency, and these generated frequencies propagate or move away from their source point. Our heart frequency, or heartbeat, is perhaps the easiest to relate to regarding this concept. We can often hear our heartbeat, especially when we are scared or have just exerted ourself. However, every part of the human body, including the brain, has its own rhythm, its own optimal frequency range. In this way the human body is like a symphony with many instruments. Ideally, everything is in tune and in harmony, but stressors can cause different parts of our being to lose their coherent frequency. Just like the way a car or an instrument can get out of tune, so can the human body. And tuning forks, by offering a coherent frequency by which the body can attune itself, offer a very simple and noninvasive way to get back "in tune."

We have been so conditioned to think of ourselves in terms of our mechanical, chemical properties that at first this notion of "frequency packets" is a little hard to conceptualize for some. But if you think about it a bit, you will come to recognize the frequency aspect of your inner composition.

So, we are almost done looking at words. I'll introduce other words as we go along and give those definitions, but before we move on let's take a look at one more term: *word*.

WHAT IS A WORD?

When we go to *Webster's* we find a dizzying array of definitions of *word*. In the interest of keeping things simple, let's just take the first one from this source, and then let's go to a more fun source: the Urban Dictionary.

Webster's: Something that is said

Urban Dictionary (online): *Word* is the shortened form of the phrase "my word is my bond," which was originated by inmates in U.S. prisons. The longer phrase was shortened to "word is bond," before becoming "word," which is most commonly used. It basically means "truth" or "to speak the truth."

In recent years this meaning of *word* as defined by the Urban Dictionary has entered the popular lexicon, beginning mainly with African American youth and then spreading into the culture at large. It is interesting to see how it relates to the Bible, which states, "In the beginning was the Word."

Now, there is not a single book on sound healing out there that does not discuss this concept: that almost all the creation stories from all over the world begin with some kind of deity speaking it into being. Our standard secular cosmological narrative takes God out of the picture, but a sound (the Big Bang) still creates something from nothing. But here is a novel way of contemplating it: say *word* aloud, very slowly, extending the *r* sound as *rrrrr* for as long as you can. What does it make you think of?

As for myself I think of an old-fashioned egg beater with two paddles, one going clockwise and the other counterclockwise, making the *rrrrr* sound. In the Vedic creation story, prana is "the word," the sound waves that arise from the luminous ocean of pure beingness, the restlessness or motion that gives rise to the ever-changing explicate reality born of the changeless implicate reality.* And so *word*—frequency—is

---

*Physicist David Bohm defined *explicate order* as the order of the external, visible, physical world and *implicate order* as the source of explicate order, an underlying whole that physical form constantly unfolds out from and enfolds back into.

motion, movement, the jitterbug dance of the two (masculine and feminine, positive and negative) arising from the one.

There is a Vedic saying, "Nada Brahma," which translates into "all is sound" or "sound is God," which means that all is brought into being by frequency, by sound. Sound provides the pattern and the motion by which all forms arise.

So, on this note, let's take a deeper look at sound.

2

SOUND— WHAT IS IT?

Understanding the Science of Sound and Why We Use It Therapeutically

> *You can look at disease as a form of disharmony.*
> *And there's no organ system in the body that's not*
> *affected by sound and music and vibration.*
>
> MITCHELL GAYNOR, M.D.,
> *SOUNDS OF HEALING*

Before we begin talking about how sound can be used therapeutically, let's talk a little bit about what it is. There are essentially two definitions of sound listed below. The first one describes vibrations within the range of human hearing, the second vibrations in general.

1. Vibrations transmitted through an elastic solid or a liquid or gas, with frequencies in the approximate range of 20 to 20,000 Hz, capable of being detected by human organs of hearing
2. Transmitted vibrations of any frequency

For the purpose of our study of Biofield Tuning, we will refer to the second definition.

Frequencies above 20,000 Hertz (abbreviated as Hz) are

referred to as *ultrasonic,* and frequencies below 20 Hz *infrasonic. Hertz* refers to cycles per second, a term named after the German physicist Heinrich Hertz (1857–1894), who made important contributions to the study of electromagnetism. For example, a 500-Hz tuning fork oscillates 500 times per second.

Frequencies produce overtones, or harmonics. A harmonic frequency is a multiple of a fundamental frequency. A fundamental frequency of 500 Hz has a first harmonic frequency of 1000 Hz (2f), double the fundamental frequency. Its second harmonic is 1500 Hz (3f), the third harmonic is 2000 Hz (4f), and so on. A musical instrument produces both fundamental tones and overtones. Technically, every tone produces

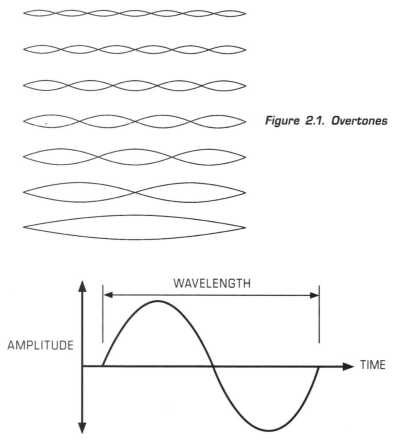

Figure 2.1. Overtones

Figure 2.2. Wavelength

infinite overtones, although we only hear the first few, a concept illustrated in figure 2.1. When we think about sound waves, we tend to think about them as depicted in the image in figure 2.2.

Figure 2.2 is the classic sine wave depiction. But in reality sound propagates spherically from its source and may travel in spiraling three-dimensional shapes. To this end I recently came across the following mind-bending description:

> For example, sound is not a vibration of the air. A sound wave, we know today, is an electromagnetic process involving the rapid assembly and disassembly of geometrical configurations of molecules. In modern physics this kind of self-organizing process is known as a "soliton." Although much more detailed experimental work needs to be done, we know in principle that different frequencies of coherent solitons correspond to distinct geometries on the microscopic or quantum level of organization of the process. This was already indicated by the work of Helmholtz's contemporary, Bernhard Riemann, who refuted most of the acoustic doctrines of Helmholtz in his 1859 paper on acoustical shock waves.[1]

In other words, rather than just the pressure wave front that we might tend to think of when we think of sound traveling (the two-dimensional sine wave that most visual depictions show), sound may actually be a complex geometric pattern moving through whatever medium it is traversing. If you have ever seen images in a cymatics video—especially those created by a CymaScope, which is a laboratory instrument that makes visible the inherent geometries within sound and music—this concept makes sense.

CYMATICS

Cymatics is the study of sound and vibration made visible through a medium such as water in a dish, or a Chladni plate, a flat metal plate on which a medium such as salt is placed, with a speaker underneath.

As the frequencies delivered through the speaker change, the geometric images produced by the frequencies also change, spontaneously and even somewhat startlingly. The higher the frequencies, the more complex the geometry produced.

The first time I saw the classic cymatics video by Hans Jenny, a Swiss medical doctor and pioneer in this field, I was stunned. I had heard the notion that "the sound current underlies all of creation," but I didn't really understand what that meant until I saw these geometric patterns appear and then disappear and then reappear completely differently in response to the sound being produced. There is one scene in particular where some iron filings resembling people dancing suddenly collapse, lifeless, when the sound is stopped, like marionettes whose strings have been cut. I highly recommend going to YouTube and looking at a variety of cymatics videos to experience this directly because it really opens your eyes (and ears) to this fascinating phenomenon.

When we see how sound affects substances, it then makes perfect sense why people chant mantras. Because humans are mostly water, any sound we produce reverberates through us, affecting all the structures in our bodies. From the tone of our voice to the words we speak and the sentiment with which we say them, the sounds we make produce a continuous creative structuring in our bodies. If you have seen Dr. Masuru Emoto's work with ice crystals, as depicted in his book *The Hidden Messages in Water,* you can see, in crystallized forms, the effects of the difference between beneficial and nonbeneficial words and intonations and how that hypothetically translates to the water in our own bodies.

Sound travels through air at approximately 350 meters per second, and through water at approximately 1500 meters per second, but this depends on many factors, including humidity and temperature. The warmer and more humid the air, the faster sound will travel through it. Generally, the denser the medium, the faster sound travels through it. For example, you can hear a train coming much sooner if you put your ear to the metal track as opposed to just listening to the air current.

COHERENT VS. INCOHERENT FREQUENCIES

Coherent is a word we use a lot in Biofield Tuning. Here's *Webster's* definition:

1. Logically or aesthetically ordered or integrated; consistent: *coherent style; a coherent argument;* having clarity or intelligibility; understandable: *a coherent person; a coherent passage*
2. Having the quality of holding together or cohering; cohesive, coordinated: *a coherent plan for action*
3. Relating to or composed of waves having a constant difference in phase: *coherent light;* producing coherent light: *a coherent source*

So, a coherent frequency is one that is ordered, consistent, clear, and in phase. *In phase* means "operating at the same frequency or wavelength." An incoherent frequency is disordered, inconsistent, not clear, and out of phase (we all know people who are coherent vs. incoherent). A tuning fork produces a coherent frequency, and that is why it is useful as a healing tool.

Research at the HeartMath Institute has found that the heart produces either coherent or incoherent frequency patterns based on the emotions a person is feeling. Feelings of love, appreciation, and gratitude cause the heart to produce coherent frequencies, whereas frustration, anger, and other so-called negative emotions cause the heart to produce incoherent frequencies.

I have had direct experience of a HeartMath technology, a simple device that measures and shows the degree of coherence produced by what is called our *heart rate variability*. HeartMath was one of the exhibitors at a conference I attended a few years ago, and I was interested to see if their technology could be useful as a biomarker measurement in my research. I sat down at the table and got hooked up to the device, a little sensor that attached to my ear, and began to chat with the representative about my research. The output on the computer screen looked like a stock market chart: it was irregular and jagged. The representative then had me think about something that gave me loving feelings, and so I mentally recalled saying good-bye to my boys before I headed out on my trip. I had to wake them up at 4 a.m. to say good-bye, and they were all sleepy and cute. As my heart swelled with this memory, the readout suddenly changed to show an orderly and balanced sine wave.

This is such a beautiful and elegant tool to show people what a difference their thoughts and feelings make regarding their health. When you consider that the heart is the driving rhythm for the entire body, and as we will see later, how every cell is bathed in its electromagnetic field, its "mood" affects the well-being of every organ and system in the body.

So, not only are we affected by the degree of coherence vs. incoherence in our inner environment, we are also affected by our outer environment.

NOISE

As I sit at my kitchen table writing this page, I am listening to my refrigerator. It is making a few different sounds: a kind of a low rumble, and then this fluctuating *wrr WRRR wrrr WRR* sound on top of that. Truly, it sounds terrible, and when I focus on it I realize that I have tension in my neck and shoulders that is bracing me against it.

I also have two fluorescent lights in the kitchen that make noise. Sometimes, if I am busy, I don't notice them, but other times I become quite aware when they are on and notice that they are making me irritable.

I once owned a restaurant, and when I worked in the kitchen there were many different noises going on all the time—the compressors in all the refrigeration units, the overhead lights, the sizzling food, the din of customer's voices, the music playing, the dishwasher running. Every once in a while, the power would go out and everything would suddenly fall silent. I always noticed that I let out a big sigh and dropped my shoulders whenever this happened. All this noise was a constant low-level stressor on my body that created muscular tension and subsequent lack of energy flow in my body. Chronic tension leads to chronic fatigue and other disorders.

The unfortunate fact of the matter is that most mechanical and electrical engines are built with little consideration as to the quality of sounds they emit as a consequence (think leaf blowers). With the exception of nuclear submarine engines and other high-performance machines, most things that run make dissonant and stressful sounds. Our modern world is so full of noise, both in our homes and outside, in such a broad spectrum of frequencies, that it's a wonder that any of us are sane or healthy. We are constantly beaten down by the chaos that surrounds us as our bodies struggle to retain the inner harmony dictated by our "factory settings," our prime frequencies.

The scientific study of the propagation, absorption, and reflection of sound waves is called *acoustics*. *Noise* is a term often used to refer to an unwanted sound. In science and engineering, noise is an undesirable component that obscures a wanted signal.

What, then, is the wanted signal? Mostly what people seem to crave as wanted signals are sounds of nature. Away from the constant din of civilization, we find restoration in nature—at the ocean, with the crashing of waves; in the forest, next to a brook's waterfall; at the top of a mountain, enjoying the silence. These kinds of sounds are often incorporated into healing music, but right now there is a growing field of practitioners and clients who are discovering the power of pure acoustic tones through the use of gongs, Tibetan and crystal singing bowls, native drums, and other acoustic instruments.

WHY USE SOUND THERAPEUTICALLY?

The human body is wired to be exquisitely sensitive to sound. The faculty of hearing is one of the first senses to develop in utero and the last to depart before death. In addition to perceiving sound through our ears, we also "hear" the pressure waves of sound through our skin, and the water that makes up approximately 70 percent of us conducts sound four to five times faster than air.

Our bones also conduct sound, as evidenced by the newer hearing aids that conduct sound through the skull directly to the cochlea, and through the technique of using a vibrating tuning fork to determine if a bone is fractured. In this technique the tuning fork is placed distal to the suspected fracture and the stethoscope is placed proximal to the injury on the same bone. A clear tone indicates an uninjured bone, whereas if the sound is diminished or absent, it indicates the presence of a fracture.[2]

It has been discovered that in addition to the traditionally viewed lock-and-key structure of receptors on cell membranes that receive and respond to physical molecules, there are also antenna-like structures (i.e., primary cilium) that respond to vibrational frequencies. Biologist Bruce Lipton writes in *The Biology of Belief:*

> Receptor antennas can also read vibrational energy fields such as light, sound, and radio frequencies. The antennas on these energy receptors vibrate like tuning forks. If an energy vibration in the environment resonates with a receptor's antenna, it will alter the protein's charge, causing the receptor to change shape. Because these receptors can read energy fields, the notion that only physical molecules can impact cell physiology is outmoded. Biological behavior can be controlled by invisible forces as well as it can be controlled by physical molecules like penicillin, a fact that provides the scientific underpinning for pharmaceutical-free energy medicine.[3]

When I first came across this passage, I had to sit and look out the window for a long time. Here was an explanation for what I had been observing for years with my tuning forks, without really understanding what was going on: teeny reciprocal tuning forks on each cell membrane, producing either incoherent or coherent frequencies, "changing their tune," as it were, when bathed in coherent sound.

This also struck me as potentially the biological mechanism of what we call intuition. We all sense "vibes" coming from other people, but *how* do we sense them? The thought of little antennas on our cells picking up ambient frequencies explains this perfectly. One of my students, a sixteen-year-old girl, told us about a wilderness program she had attended where one of their exercises was to walk blindfolded through the forest while some of their fellow students hid and broadcast ill intentions. The process was designed to sensitize the students to pick up on these frequencies.

This is how all of nature operates, by paying attention to these kinds of signals. Any of us who have pets know that pets can read our vibes without having to use words. And research into plants has shown that they too can read our vibes. In *The Secret Life of Plants*, author Peter Tompkins recounts how he hooks some plants up to a polygraph machine and discovers, among many other interesting things, that the plants register alarm when he has the intention of burning them with matches.

I had a memorable experience last summer with tuning forks and plants hooked up to a polygraph machine (no matches were involved). I was visiting some friends in Colorado, and we went to visit one of their friends, Luiz, who was conducting Ph.D. research at the University of Colorado in a manner similar to the work of Tompkins. He had two different plants in his lab, attached by thin metal probes to a polygraph system in his computer. We wanted to see how the plants would respond to "getting a tune-up."

I began, like I do with my clients, by locating the edge of the field, which was about 2.5 feet away from the plant itself, slowly working my way in toward it. Almost immediately, the polygraph readout began to edge downward. "That means the plant is relaxing," Luiz told me. The readout continued its downward descent as I moved in closer and closer to the plant. And then a curious thing happened. In Biofield Tuning there is a lightening or brightening of the tone once the work on any given chakra is complete—a sort of release of the process. I sensed this happening with the plant, but then returned with another strike of the fork anyway, and immediately the readout began to edge back upward. The plant seemed to know its treatment was complete and began to resist my continued advances.

The next plant provided another very curious experience. While the first one was an Amazonian medicinal plant, this second plant was just a regular ornamental bamboo house plant. As I approached it with the fork, the readout on the computer hardly changed at all; if anything, it edged upward slightly, and what I encountered was something that I absolutely had not anticipated: the fork was reflecting in its overtones the frequency signature that I have come to recognize in people as fear, with a pulsing quality to the sound. It appeared that the poor plant was afraid of me! I said this to Luiz, and he replied, "It is interesting that you say that because I actually had a very good psychic here last week, a woman who works with the Colorado State Police, and she also told me that the plant was afraid." The implications of this were profound—it appeared that there was a common emotional vibrational language not just among people and animals, but with flora as well. This explained how and why Tompkin's plants sensed his intention to harm them. It also made me think of how we say "dogs smell fear," and while they no doubt do, they also sense fear, along with every other vibrational emotion we are emitting, because we all speak the same language on the level of our vibes.

Before we go much further exploring how and why sound works on the body, let's answer a question that I am often asked: How did I get into sound in the first place?

3

HOW BIOFIELD TUNING CAME TO BE

My Journey of Learning to Sing, Discovering the Biofield, and Sharing My Practice

Does the walker choose the path, or the path the walker?

GARTH NIX, *SABRIEL*

It was never my intention to be a sound healer. But sometimes life has a way of guiding us into things, whether we think we want to go that way or not. My journey has progressed, like a trail of crumbs, from one book to the next, one workshop and wellness practice to another, and has led me to where I am now, with an unusual viewpoint that I had no idea I would find when I first set off on my journey.

My path has been one of healing, and it first emerged when I was eighteen years old. I was bulimic, and had been for over a year. It started innocently enough, when I was working at a pizza parlor and also going to modeling school. I loved and wanted to eat pizza, but the weigh-in at school each week made it clear that if I wanted to have anything to do with modeling, I definitely needed to be skinnier. One day one of my coworkers said to me, "I know how you can eat whatever you want and not gain weight. Just stick your finger down your throat after each meal." I had heard of bulimia. I knew that there had been some girls in my high school who did it, but it had truly never occurred to me to do it myself until this moment. It certainly seemed to solve my problem, so I decided to give it a try.

This simple acquiescence led me into three years of binge-and-purge hell. On the outside I was pretty, confident, and highly functional, but on the inside I became a mess of constant obsession about what I was going to eat where and when, and how I was going to hide throwing it back up again. After the first year, I confessed to my mother, who had grown up in Belfast, Northern Ireland, during World War II and had never had enough to eat. She was skinny as a rail and always had been. She made an attempt to help me by scheduling an appointment for me with the doctor who was covered by her HMO at the time, saying, "I don't understand this. This is a disease of your time."

In my visit with this doctor, I got into an argument with him over whether reality was subjective or objective: he insisted there was an objective reality; I insisted that the process of observing and defining it rendered reality subjective, and after a few minutes of debate, he threw up his hands and exclaimed, "I cannot help you!"

After that I was on my own. And so I started to search for answers to my questions: "Why can I not stop doing this?" "How is it that I have lost control of myself?" "How do I stop my brain from running constantly with this torturous inner dialogue?" "How do I get a grip?" "What is wrong with me?"

Up until this point I had always been a nerdy kid: braces, glasses, nose buried in a book. As a little girl I never had what I call the "pretty girl syndrome" because I had always identified with my braininess. I had skipped two grades and graduated from a prestigious prep school when I was just sixteen. But that summer after graduation, after the braces came off and the glasses gave way to contacts, I suddenly realized I didn't look half bad, and just for the heck of it I ended up entering the Miss Teen Connecticut pageant. Much to my amazement, I won runner-up and also the Miss Photogenic award. Suddenly, I was pretty. And while this boosted my self-esteem, it came with an unanticipated downside: being a pretty girl meant being skinny. I wasn't really skinny. I had big bones, thick wrists and ankles, wide feet, and a propensity toward solid rather than slender. I had worked to lose a few pounds for the competition (and lied about my weight besides), but now I felt a pressure I had never felt before to really look and play the part. *Vogue* and *Mademoiselle* magazines piled up next to my bedside table, and makeup and shoes and clothes consumed the money I made waitressing.

When the bulimia started, I was five-foot-six and weighed about 130 pounds, which according to standard height/weight charts is the ideal weight for a woman. But I had it in my head, as encouraged by the fashion magazines I could not seem to put down, that I should weigh 115 or even less. And so I began to obsess about my weight, weighing myself multiple times a day and beating myself up if the needle edged upward from my ideal. It didn't take long for this to morph into full-blown obsessive-compulsive behavior, and by the time I started purging, I had already been binge eating. Ultimately, the bulimia didn't make me lose weight; it just stopped me from gaining any. It was a tortuous cycle that led nowhere.

So when I was eighteen, after the failed visit to the family doctor, I picked up my first self-help book: *TNT: The Power Within You.* After years of reading fiction voraciously, I now turned that ability to inhale books toward everything I could find in the self-help category. This expanded outward to science and spirituality, health and wellness, and human potential. I read Edgar Cayce, Carlos Castenada, Tony Robbins, Wayne Dyer, Marianne Williamson, Deepak Chopra, Louise Hay, Carolyn Myss, and so many more. As a result, two very key points dawned on me. The first was the realization that I had been programmed into my self-destructive behavior. Our culture holds up two signs to women: Consume, and Be Skinny. I had managed to figure out a way to do both. I wasn't controlling enough to become anorexic, and I wasn't so out of control as to be obese. In classic Libra form, I had figured out how to reconcile opposites.

Realizing that I was responding to programming helped take the sting out of the shame of "What is wrong with me?" but it didn't impact my behavior right away. What finally got me to stop the binge-and-purge behavior was the second realization—that it was my hand and my mouth, and if I wasn't in control, then who was? I saw that I needed to accept responsibility for my choices and find it within myself to step into the cycle of behavior and break it.

By the time I was twenty, I had stopped throwing up, but the binge-ing was not so easy to stop. To complicate matters considerably, I had opened a café with my family that year. This was preceded by an eight-month solo backpacking trip through Europe before my nineteenth birthday, after which I found myself trying to figure out what to do with my life. Having gone to Europe to find myself, I had accomplished just that, to some degree. I realized that I was a writer after finding myself, pen in hand, scribbling furiously in notebooks in cafés all over Europe. But I also realized that I had nothing meaningful to write about yet, that I needed some water under the bridge before writing could bear fruit in my life. Meanwhile, I needed to occupy myself.

One day, while out on a walk shortly after returning from Europe, the proverbial flash of inspiration lit up my brain: the idea of the Vanilla Bean Café came to me, fully formed. My nickname all my life had been Bean. As the youngest of six kids, and then the youngest and smallest in my class at school, the name had stuck, and not one person called me by my given name, Eileen. I was so excited by the idea that I ran the last mile home, to the building that my parents had bought while I was in Europe and that they had moved their mail-order business into.

"Mom, Dad, let's open up a café in the other half of the building!" I said, breathlessly. They agreed, on the spot. It wasn't really that much of a bolt from the blue. We were a family of foodies. My mother was a famously great cook, and I had made my first restaurant menu when I was just seven years old. (I still have it, actually. It has, among other strange things, escargot as an appetizer.) The building was in a great location for such an enterprise. It was an old carriage barn that had once been attached to a grand home that had burned down, located on a corner in town, with plenty of parking, and had already had several incarnations as different businesses.

My mother recruited two of my four older brothers to help, and after jumping through all kinds of hoops to get it open, "the Bean," as it became known, opened in Pomfret, Connecticut, in August 1989 with sixteen seats and just the four of us at the helm. We had soups and sandwiches, espresso drinks, baked goods, desserts (oh my, did we have desserts!), ice cream, and a frozen yogurt machine. My mother made quiche, my brothers made soups and chili, and I did all of the baking.

To say that the first few years of the Vanilla Bean were stressful for me would be a huge understatement. Within four years we had, including outside seating, 140 seats and over thirty employees. We had nonstop construction going on, bumping our half of the building into another third, and then finally booting the mail-order business out altogether, as well as putting on a large addition in the back that doubled the size of the kitchen.

In the first year, I worked from six in the morning until ten at night almost every single day. I did all the baking in the morning, worked every meal, and then mopped the floors at night, only to get up and do it all over again the next day and the day after that. And while we grew and grew like mad, there were long stretches during the day, especially during the winter, when there were no customers to wait on. During these times I endured a furious inner battle: Brownie? Carrot cake? Lemon poppy-seed muffin? Chocolate mousse cake? Ice cream?

The stress of the business, the customers, my older brothers, the employees, and the relentless hours broke down my willpower, and my weight ballooned up to 170 pounds. This might not sound like a lot, but to a teen beauty queen it was a fate worse than death. I was incapable of eating properly and simply grazed through every day, eating sugar, flour, chocolate, dairy, and coffee. My adrenals became more and more taxed, my nerves became more and more frayed, until it finally dawned on me that I was killing myself and that I needed to stop.

I had kept on reading nonfiction books and realized that in my quest for personal wellness I had developed an interest in natural medicine. I considered going to school to become a naturopath but wasn't that keen on going back to school for the twelve years or whatever it was going to take to do that. I ended up deciding instead to leave the café and go to massage therapy school in Cambridge, Massachusetts.

It was extremely difficult to leave the café. My brothers were not happy at all with my decision. I felt extremely guilty for coming up with the idea, roping everyone into it, putting us all through an epic struggle, and then splitting the scene. But there was no getting around the fact that I was a wreck: my back, in fact, was completely wrecked from standing over the sink, over the sandwich bar, over the stove, over the mop bucket. I was in constant, chronic pain. I also was suffering from acute TMJ that would send shooting pains up into my ears at random times. My cholesterol was over 220, my adrenals were burned out, and I was overly emotional about just about everything.

Massage school seemed like a good antidote to all of that, plus an opportunity to begin an education in the field of health and wellness. And it was. I got a job waitressing at the House of Blues in Harvard Square and an apartment in Somerville and effortlessly dropped to a size four. I ate regular meals, rode my bike to work, enjoyed the atmosphere at school, and started going to yoga classes. I also received ten Rolfing sessions (a form of deep bodywork that creates a greater degree of structural integration). I got healthy, in shape, and happier.

But come February I began to feel the depression creep in again. It wasn't just the food that had been the problem, I realized; I had been suffering from depression to varying degrees since I was seventeen or so. It was worse in the winter, but it came at other times as well. I continued to suffer from depression, from that heavy feeling that something is sitting on your heart, until I had my first son at age twenty-nine. And then it stopped, like magic. It probably was hormonal, but I also think it was because when Quinn was born I had to stop thinking about myself so much. It was all my thinking about myself and my woes that had made me feel depressed, the stories I was telling myself. Suddenly, I had someone else to think about and something important to do full-time, and the dysfunctional, depressed, food- and weight-obsessed nonsense all just sort of disappeared. It also helped that I had been doing and then teaching yoga for a couple of years before I got pregnant. Yoga had helped me tremendously in my quest to eat better and feel better about my body, by, among other things, putting me back in touch with my "I'm full" switch that years of bingeing had caused me to override and disable.

But prior to that, and even in the years subsequent to that, winter, especially February, really found me down in the dumps. In hindsight it's easy to see that a significant part of my suffering was a vitamin D deficiency. Now I know that taking a few thousand IUs of vitamin D3 during the winter months can do wonders, but back in 1995 I had no idea. All I knew was the familiar feeling of depression and stagnation was returning after many months of it being completely gone. And then I got a fateful phone call that changed everything. My mother, who had never asked for help, was on the other end crying and telling me that she needed help, that she had developed symptoms that seemed to indicate she had suffered a stroke.

My mother was diagnosed with a glioblastoma, the most aggressive type of brain tumor, which doubles in size every thirty to sixty days. It was already the size of a lemon and pressing on the part of her brain that controlled speech and fine motor skills by the time we saw the CT scan. We chose surgery, but it made it far worse: the surgeon told us she would live perhaps six months, but she was dead within six weeks, and I suddenly found myself back in Pomfret, filling my mother's impossibly big shoes.

My mother had been a pillar of the community who ran two businesses and took care of my handicapped father full-time. My father had had a massive stroke when he was fifty-nine and I was ten. It had left him completely paralyzed on his right side, and in the beginning it took away his speech completely. Through rehab, he had learned to walk with a cane and speak again, but he always struggled with word retrieval. He had no problem cursing or singing, though. My mother had been taking care of him ever since then—every day for the last sixteen years. She got him up, dressed and fed him, and brought him to work, where he would type with his one good hand. She bathed him and put him in pajamas and into bed every night. We all thought that at some point Dad would die and Mom would get her life back. None of us ever dreamed that Mom would go first.

So there I was, suddenly, back in the restaurant, and now taking care of my father and the mail-order business to boot. But I had learned a few things at massage school about boundaries, about self-care, and I was determined to not dissolve back into the restaurant, but to maintain my interest in and pursuit of the healing arts.

LEARNING TO SING

I started doing a few massages a week, and also returned to taking singing lessons. When I was twenty I had received very clear inner guidance that I was to learn how to sing. I had never had a good singing voice. I was the kid in music class who clapped on the off-beat, sang off-key, and squeaked my clarinet. I was decidedly nonmusical and even ashamed of my voice. But there it was, that insistent guidance that never stopped nudging (that "subtle magnetism" of Thoreau, or what I later came to call the "mail slot") until I acted on it. I booked my first appointment and went to it with my heart in my throat. The music teacher played middle C on the piano over and over, trying to get me to match the tone with a *la*. I could not make a sound. My knees shook and my palms sweated until I finally choked out a strangled noise and then burst into tears.

Over the next seven years, I went to seven different voice teachers. The first five told me I would never be able to sing because I was tone deaf: I could not hear the notes clearly and replicate them properly and was forever singing off-key. However, I couldn't get the African proverb "If you can walk, you can dance; if you can talk, you can sing" out of my mind. It seemed to me a human birthright to be able to sing, and I was convinced I could, that everyone could; I just needed to find the right teacher.

I spent many a lesson coming home in tears, wondering what on earth was wrong with me, or what had happened to me that I was so incredibly bound up inside. Many of my lessons felt like torture, but I kept on going back, again and again. By the time I had made it to the sixth teacher, I had made some small strides but still was off-key most of the time. What was different about my sixth teacher, aside from the fact that she believed we could get somewhere, was the fact that in this time period I had started doing yoga and had gone through the ten sessions of Rolfing. The patterns of tension in my body that were reflected in my voice began to loosen and soften.

I had spent most of my childhood in a defensive mode. As the youngest of six, with six to twelve years between me and the rest of the pack, I was both vulnerable and sensitive (according to my mother, I was "overly sensitive" and "took everything to heart") and was constantly fending off things like Indian rope burn, tickle attacks, "the claw," camel bites, and biting sarcasm. Skipping two grades in school had also put me at the bottom of the pecking order there, and I came home in tears many days from the sheer cruelty I endured from being so much littler and geekier than everyone else. (I didn't finally hit a growth spurt and stop looking like I was in sixth grade until I was sixteen and a senior in high school.)

And from age ten on, after my father had his stroke, my parents, who had never before been a source of stress to me, now were a source of constant stress. After his stroke my father started suffering grand mal seizures that were unpredictable, scary, and violent, and even after they were brought under control with medication he would occasionally cut back on it without telling us because he didn't like having to take drugs. This would inevitably lead to another unanticipated and alarming seizure.

My mother suffered a nervous breakdown after my father's stroke. She had always been patient, dependable, and loving toward me. Now, overwhelmed by suddenly being saddled with a severely handicapped husband, plus the responsibilities of handling my father's business (which due to the inflation of the '70s was running in the red for the first time in its long history), maintaining a large home, caring for four teenage children (most of whom were prone to drinking and driving), and me at age ten, Mother began pacing the halls at night, screaming that she wished she were dead. I moved my bed into her room to stop her screaming at night, and it worked. But before that thought occurred to me I would lie in bed in my room, holding my breath, every muscle taut as a piano wire. I wished fervently that my father would get better and that the nightmare would end, and though he recovered somewhat, he would thereafter always require constant care.

So all of these experiences combined to make me bound up inside, creating an armored physiology. Once, when talking with my husband about this, I said that I was "well defended," to which he replied, "You're not well defended; you're supremely fortified."

It has been my observation in my practice that the more intelligent a person is, the more elaborate their defenses, both in shielding from unpleasant memories within and from unpleasant stimuli without. I had constructed an elaborate defense system in order to cope with the constant barrage of stress, and it involved locking down a great many places in my body. Brain signals responsible for larynx movement travel through the vagus nerve, also called the "wandering nerve" because it travels throughout much of the body. When there is constriction in the body, this is reflected in the voice. We all know how easy it is to tell when someone is under stress when we hear their voice on the phone; the physical constriction contracts the nervous system and it is reflected in the tonal quality of the voice. Additionally, in Chinese medicine, the kidneys "open to the ears." They are also said to hold the vibrations of shock and fear. My kidneys have always been a weak link, and various energy medicine practitioners have alluded to blocked energy in my kidneys. This no doubt played a role in my hearing deficiency as well.

So, during the time that I was working with my sixth voice teacher, I experienced a number of breakthroughs that allowed me to relax enough to hear more clearly and to start to be able to sing on-key with more regularity. I still felt bound, like I had a knot in my throat, but at least I was getting somewhere. By the time I got to my seventh teacher, she said, after our first practice together, "You can hear and sing fine." It was such an enormous relief to finally hear those words! So, based on this experience I believe that it is possible for most people who do not have an actual physical shortcoming with their auditory system to learn how to sing. It may take a ridiculous amount of perseverance, but tone-deafness does not have to be a life sentence.

Today, people tend to be surprised to discover that I had to learn how to hear, and that I am not naturally musical, though there seems to be a general assumption that I am. I have found that while I have the patience to teach that which was difficult for me to learn, I have very little patience teaching what comes easily to me. (A baking lesson from me goes something like, "You throw some of this in with some of this, mix it together and leave it in the oven until it smells done.") Being able to hear clearly is something I had to work very hard at.

And I definitely don't have perfect pitch—even after using the C scale of tuning forks for fifteen years, I cannot identify which note is being played if someone picks a random fork and activates it. I've always focused more on the information in the overtones than the actual sound of the note itself, which may have something to do with this. That said, from the first time I picked up tuning forks, I could "hear the stories" in the dissonance of the overtones as they passed over the body. Which brings us to this part of our story: how the process I call *Biofield Tuning* began and evolved.

HOW BIOFIELD TUNING CAME TO BE

I am a researcher by nature, and when I become interested in a particular subject, I tend to read everything I can find on it. In 1996 someone gave me a book on the use of color and sound in healing. This was shortly after I had come across quantum physics and the notion that everything is vibration. It appeared to me at once that if everything is vibration, then treating vibration with vibration is logical and elegant, and so I proceeded to read everything I could find on this subject. As I was getting to the end of my stack, I received a catalog in the mail advertising a set of "tuning forks for healing," which I ordered on impulse. The tuning forks were called the Solar Harmonic Spectrum set: eight forks in the octave of the C major scale. They came with very simple directions: use the note of C over the root chakra, the note of D over the sacral chakra, and so on, up to the note of B at the crown chakra. According to the Vedic and other ancient traditions, there are seven major energy centers, or chakras, that run along the spine; these are considered part of the body's subtle anatomy.

I began experimenting with the tuning forks with a few of my massage therapy clients. I activated the forks by striking them against a hockey puck and then held them over the body as instructed. I immediately noticed that the quality of the sound—the volume, pitch, and timbre—changed, depending on where the tuning fork was held. This was very surprising to me, as I expected the fork to produce a steady, regular tone. A single strike could produce tones that were flat, sharp, dull, loud, soft, or full of static as I moved the fork around the body.

Furthermore, I found that if a client was complaining of pain in a particular area, the fork would produce either a loud, sharp tone or a tone full of static and "noise." After holding the fork over the area, perhaps six inches or so over the body, I found that after a few moments the tone would become clear. Again, much to my surprise, the client would return the following week and tell me that all her pain was gone after the session. People also reported to me that they felt more calm, clear, and "lighter" after sessions.

Another curious phenomenon that I observed was that I could actually "drag around" the spots that were more energized, which I assumed was the case in areas where the tone became louder. For example, if I passed the tuning fork over a person's hip and the tone became louder there, I could do what felt like "hooking in" to the energized area, and pull it along with the fork. It made sense to me that it should sound loud down the center of the body, along the spine, at the areas where the chakras and the nerve plexi are located.

I developed a technique that I called "click, drag, and drop," which is essentially a "combing" of what I can only describe as energy from the periphery of the body to the vertical midline. The process felt akin to using a magnet to move iron filings across a surface. I noticed a definite increase in the volume of the fork in the area over each chakra after I completed this dragging process.

Chakras

The word *chakra* means "wheel," and these energy centers are considered spinning wheels or vortexes of subtle energy flow. As one can see in figure 3.1 on page 56, these centers sit approximately in the same places as our nerve plexi (think of subtle energy as a higher harmonic of the electricity present in a nerve cluster).

I don't really like using the word *chakra* because it is one of those words that for many people has the charge of the unknown. In my effort to bridge the domains of science and spirituality, I try, whenever possible, to choose words or phrases that are more familiar. There is no English equivalent of the word *chakra,* however, because the concept of this feature of our energy anatomy does not exist in English.

Clients began requesting that I use sound more and more, and within a few months I found myself doing more sound sessions than straight massage sessions. Since I was in brand-new territory, with no real road map other than the simple instructions the forks came with, I had to trust my senses and my intuitive guidance as I moved forward with the process.

THE MAIL SLOT

The mail slot is the metaphor I use for describing intuitive guidance. I came across this concept once in a book, the title of which I cannot remember, wherein the author was discussing his experience of the intuitive process. He described it as a mail slot in the back of his head that would randomly open and a note would drop in. He found that if the note contained instructions to do something, for example, and he did it, he would observe a beneficial outcome. As a result, he had learned to trust and follow whatever came in through the mail slot.

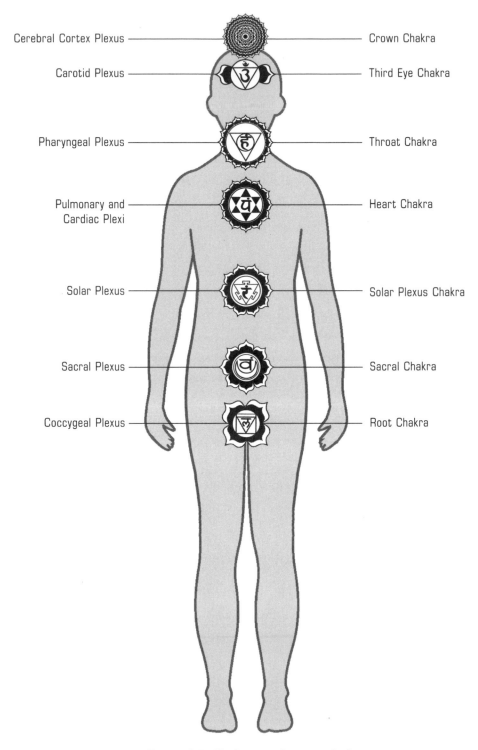

Cerebral Cortex Plexus ——————————— Crown Chakra

Carotid Plexus ——————————— Third Eye Chakra

Pharyngeal Plexus ——————————— Throat Chakra

Pulmonary and ——————————— Heart Chakra
Cardiac Plexi

Solar Plexus ——————————— Solar Plexus Chakra

Sacral Plexus ——————————— Sacral Chakra

Coccygeal Plexus ——————————— Root Chakra

Figure 3.1. Chakras and nerve plexi

I think this is a great way to describe what we call inner guidance, or the inner teacher, and as someone who has been self-taught in the use of tuning forks, I would say that this has been my experience as well. I become uncomfortable when people talk about things like guides, whether angelic, animal, or otherwise, because from my perspective we really can't know what is behind this information drop. And I for one am content with this mystery.

I bring up the mail slot here because it was really this process that informed so much of how this work developed. Perhaps it is because of the way I was raised. After having five kids, with me being the youngest, my parents had figured out a few things and gave me a lot of room to "do what you feel like doing." Consequently, I've always been very attuned to my inner awareness. I also traveled extensively by myself between the ages of seventeen and twenty and had to rely completely on my own awareness and intuition to navigate this process. Because of all this, I don't suffer the fear, doubt, and uncertainty that many people experience when it comes to hearing and trusting their inner guidance.

DISCOVERING THE ENERGY FIELD AROUND THE BODY

I continued using the simple click, drag, and drop method on the seven major chakras on the front of the body until one day I got the idea to flip a person over and go down the back. I was surprised to discover a completely different terrain in the back and began to incorporate that into each session.

My biggest breakthrough with the work, however, occurred one day in 2005, quite by accident. I was approaching the table with the tuning fork activated (usually I activated the fork right next to the body), when about two and a half feet to the side of the client's throat the tone of the fork flared up and became quite loud and sharp. I investigated the area and discovered a "pocket" about four inches wide that, when the fork passed through it, the volume went up. When the fork passed out of it, the volume went back down. Intrigued, I employed the click, drag, and drop technique, tugging the pocket back to the throat chakra, where it felt as though it was literally sucked into the body. This particular client had been complaining of jaw, neck, and shoulder pain on that side. When I had initially investigated the area I was surprised to find no noise over it, and was puzzling over this observation when I discovered that the noise was in fact out in the client's energy field, which is what I had surmised based on what I had read in esoteric literature up to that point.

This person had gone to many different kinds of practitioners, including an osteopath, an acupuncturist, a chiropractor, and a massage therapist, and had found no relief from this uncomfortable condition. She called me the day after the session to tell me that, much to her surprise (and mine), the pain was completely gone. And it stayed gone after that, returning only briefly and occasionally when she was under stress.

After this, I began to explore the area around the body. I went as far off to the side as space allowed—about six feet—and from there combed my way in on the plane of the treatment table toward the body. I began to find phenomena I perceived as "pockets" and "walls" and "fields" and different kinds of vibrational information expressed through the overtones on every person I worked on, in various positions all around the body. I found that I seemed to have the ability to translate the feedback or "hear the story" that the forks were sending. (This ability to hear more than the average person is called *clairaudience,* as contrasted with *clairvoyance,* which describes the phenomenon of seeing more, as in the case of seeing colors in people's energy fields.) In certain areas the tone would sound or feel sad, or angry, or fearful, or any number of different emotions. Much like how a minor third in music is a universal expression of sadness, the interface between what seemed to me to be a pattern of information stored in the field and the sound of the tuning forks evoked a sense of emotion, just as music does. And much to my surprise (this work has surprised and continues to surprise me regularly), I began to find that the same emotions seem to reside in the same places in each person.

For example, I kept observing, or more precisely, hearing, the emotion of sadness in the area off the left shoulder, the emotions of guilt or shame in the area off the right hip, a sense of worry off the left side of the head, and so on, throughout the body. It took a few years, but, like putting together a puzzle, the entire picture of what I now call the *biofield anatomy* emerged. I'll go into detail about the biofield anatomy in chapter 7.

Very often when I found a pocket of energy and information, I could "hear," via the mail slot, not only what the emotion involved was, but also the age at which it was first generated. I noticed that information generated currently or in the recent past was closer to the body, while information from earliest childhood, including even gestation and birth, was at the outer edge of the field, which is about five feet out on most people, with the rest of the life history falling in between, like tree rings. These observations were inconsistent with the traditional esoteric literature, where I found nothing like a description of this time-line phenomenon, or compartmentalization of specific emotions in specific places off to the sides of the chakras. While much of what I found was in line with Carolyn Myss's description of the emotions that reside *in* each chakra, found in her book *Anatomy of the Spirit,* I had otherwise found no other references to this particular phenomenon, despite having read extensively on the subject. This being the case, I proceeded tentatively with the notion that what I was observing was an objective phenomenon. Only after seeing the patterns repeat over and over again, in many hundreds of people, and now having my students observe the same phenomenon, do I now feel more confident that this structure of information storage may in fact exist within the body's energy field, at least on the level of the energy field that interfaces with the audible frequencies produced by the forks.

That said, I want to point out that the possibility also exists that this may be a construct of my imagination. A client of mine who is a dowser and teaches dowsing told me a story about how in one of his classes he had constructed an Earth energy line with his mind in a particular place in the field behind his house. He instructed his students that this line was present there somewhere, but did not tell them

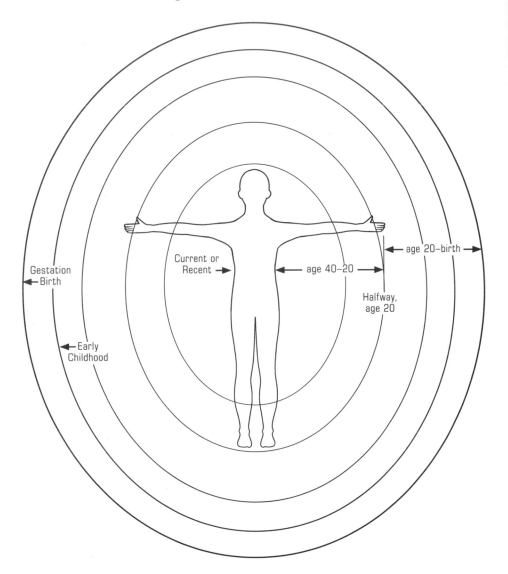

Figure 3.2. Age rings of the biofield for a forty-year-old person.
Similar to tree rings, the record of our early years moves outward,
away from the body, as we age
Illustration by Kimberly Lipinski

that he had constructed it with his imagination. Subsequently they all went back there and found it with their dowsing rods. He then deconstructed it with his mind, after which none of his students could find it anymore. The mind is very powerful and capable of things far beyond what we have been taught. This example provides evidence that this entire structure that I call the *biofield anatomy* may exist only as a construct that seems to appear when I am working on people, and is not, in fact, really there.

A small experiment I conducted points to this possibility. I was demonstrating the technique to a physics professor who suggested I try holding the fork with a clamp instead of my hand to see what happened. I was stunned to find that the volume change that I had come to rely on as an indication that I was encountering "energy" or "charge" did not occur when I was not touching the fork with my hands. I could hear the changes in the overtones, but the volume produced by the fork remained consistent as it passed through the field. This shows me that my energy is clearly influencing the process, as using the clamp interrupts the circuit of energy exchange. So when it comes right down to it, I don't *really* understand what is happening, and it is because of this not knowing that I wish to continue my research, making use of sensitive recording equipment and possibly a mechanical arm and self-striking tuning fork. Although as my students have pointed out, regardless of whether the biofield is truly and objectively there or not, the method and structure can be taught, replicated, and produces beneficial outcomes, regardless.

COMMITTING TO SOUND

In 2006 I reached an interesting crossroads with my practice. I had been doing it part-time, through word of mouth, for ten years, seeing at most two to three people a week. It was a curiosity, a hobby, but nothing I had any desire to do as a vocation. For one thing I had a very hard time reconciling my inner capitalist with my inner healer—the two just didn't seem to go together. And then there was the fact that the practice was strange and difficult to explain. It seemed a lot easier to just keep it as an occasional hobby.

I had sold my part of the Vanilla Bean to my brothers in 2002 after The Coca-Cola Company surprised us by choosing the Vanilla Bean

Café to be the launch site of Coca-Cola Vanilla. Apparently, in seeking to do something outside the box for this launch, they had done an internet search of the word *vanilla* and came across our website. In May 2002 the first cases of vanilla Coke were delivered to the Vanilla Bean Café in Pomfret, Connecticut, briefly turning it into what the media called "the soft drink center of the universe." Subsequently, we were featured in every major New England newspaper, and for several weeks it was the only place where you could buy vanilla Coke. Our already busy restaurant now swarmed with people, and I used the opportunity to bow out completely and turn the business over to my brothers. Since our father had died in 1998 after three years of our caring for him, I had nothing to keep me in Pomfret, and my husband and I decided to fulfill our dream of living in Vermont.

We settled in a town called Johnson, in the northern part of the state, and after a few years of living simply, working part-time jobs and enjoying my boys, who were one and four when we moved, I felt the entrepreneurial itch to start another business. Because I already had experience with food but didn't want to get back into the restaurant business, I decided to create some kind of specialty food company. I went to grocery stores on Sunday evenings and looked at the kinds of products that had been "hit"—that had sold more than others. I was looking for an unfilled niche, an up-and-coming market, and a good profit margin.

The idea to make kettle corn (popcorn that is both sweet and salty) came to me one day while I was in my kitchen trying to come up with a snack for the boys. I had actually never eaten kettle corn, but I had seen people stand in long lines for it at fairs and festivals, and I had never seen it anywhere in a store. So I immediately set out to start a kettle-corn business. I got a commercial kettle-corn kettle, some ingredients, and started whipping up batches of the stuff. Since I was in Vermont, it made sense to make it maple, and since I was oriented that way, I also made it organic. I started bringing samples around to local stores, and within a relatively short time I was supplying over fifty stores, some of them large grocery stores.

After less than two years, I reached a juncture with the popcorn where doing it by hand had become unwieldy. It was flying off the shelves and demand kept growing, and as a result my original infrastructure could not keep up. I needed to expand and automate to some extent, but I did not have the resources to do it on my own, and so I required investors. I put together a business plan and began to seek assistance, but kept running into roadblocks. It began to feel as if the universe was dropping boulders in my path until one day I finally stopped and said, "If something is meant to happen, it happens. This is not happening, so maybe something else is supposed to happen, in which case I am open to whatever that is."

Sometimes I get mail slot drops that are like certified mail as opposed to Post-it Notes. The idea for the Vanilla Bean Café, the thought to move to Vermont—mail drops for key turning points like these come with a certain extra wattage to them. A few days after questioning the wisdom of trying to power through the obstacles I was encountering, I received very clear guidance from the mail slot: "The world needs harmony more than it needs another snack food. Sell the popcorn business as it is, go to school, get some degrees, and learn and teach about sound." How could I argue with that?

This was a Friday morning. That day I ran into an acquaintance and ended up having lunch with her. She asked me how things were going with my popcorn business, and I told her that I was planning on selling it, that I was going to run some ads the following week. She was the only person I told this to besides my husband. Two days later she ran into an acquaintance of hers at the grocery store and my name came up. He asked her how things were going in my popcorn business and she informed him that I was planning on running some ads to sell it. "Oh, don't let her do that!" he told her. "I would be very interested in buying it!"

And he did. Six weeks later, in November 2006, I sold the popcorn business to him, enrolled in a few classes at the Community College of Vermont, and committed to seeing more clients. Over the next few years I would finish both my undergraduate and graduate degrees and end up growing a busy practice both as a practitioner and a teacher of the Biofield Tuning method, including teaching a class on sound healing at Northern Vermont University.

MY FIRST SOLFEGGIO FORKS

In 2008 I added a new set of forks to my practice, a nine-piece, unweighted Solfeggio set. Generally, unweighted forks are used over the body, and weighted forks, with small weights attached to the ends of the tines, are used with the handles placed directly on the body. This set has clearer and brighter tones than the C-scale set, and though it is not technically a musical scale, I use it in the same ascending fashion, with the lower tones on the lower part of the body and the higher tones on the upper part.

It's an interesting story as to how I ended up choosing the Solfeggio forks. I had started to feel like I needed a new and different set of forks, and so I went online to see what was available. There were so many different sets that I became confused about what to choose. I've developed the habit when I am confused of asking the universe for some kind of sign, and have found it to be a helpful practice, and this experience was no different. About a week after my request, I received an email from an acquaintance, who wrote to me, "I met a woman yesterday who uses Solfeggio tuning forks. Have you ever heard of them?" To which I replied that I hadn't, but thanked him for sharing. About a week after this, I got another email from a friend of mine who had been watching YouTube videos: "I just saw a video about Solfeggio tuning forks—have you heard of them?" To which I replied, "Why, yes, in fact, I have heard of them."

And about a week after this, I met a girlfriend for lunch. We sat down at a table and she pulled a book out of her bag and handed it to me. "As I was leaving the house, this book practically jumped off the shelf at me. I think you're supposed to read it." The book was titled *Healing Codes for the Biological Apocalypse,* by Leonard Horowitz and Joseph Puleo, and as I discovered upon reading it, it was the story of how the Solfeggio scale, as represented in the tuning fork sets I had been hearing about, came to be.

Seeing as how this was the third time in three weeks that I had heard about this scale, and seeing as how the scale is based on the number 3, I took that as a solid indication that my next set of tuning forks should probably be the Solfeggio set. When it arrived I was so enchanted by the beauty of the tones—they are clear, crystalline, and bright—that I immediately abandoned the Solar Harmonic Spectrum, which sounded dull and muddy in comparison. I used this set solely for a while but found that in some cases, especially when someone was in any kind of acute situation, the tones, when being in a part of the field that sharpened the tone, were actually too bright, and so I ended up using both sets together in sessions until the end of 2012, when I stopped using the Harmonic Spectrum altogether.

MORE ADDITIONS TO MY REPERTOIRE

In 2008 I began to work on people's feet. For some reason I did not get any clear information around people's feet regarding what resistance in that area might relate to, and I never really have to date. They remain a bit of a mystery to me and are a blank area in the biofield anatomy map. Then in 2009 I began to incorporate work on people's knees. I found the information contained in the knees—regarding forward movement, release, and spontaneous action—to be so key to a person's ability to become "unstuck" (think "knee-jerk reaction") that I was somewhat mortified that I had been doing the sound work for so long without incorporating this critical part of the anatomy.

Even without this piece, though, I had been continually receiving fascinating feedback from people regarding their experiences with the work. The sound appeared particularly useful for pain and anxiety; in some cases I heard that massive anxiety disorders had resolved in just one session, or that pain a person had experienced for thirty years was gone the morning after the first session. Clients told me it was helpful for many other kinds of issues as well: digestive disorders, menstrual disorders, depression, insomnia, migraines, emotional "stuckness," fibromyalgia, arthritis, and much more.

Although I had been using a weighted C128 fork occasionally for a few years, mostly by placing the handle on shoulder knots, in 2010 I acquired a weighted 26-Hz fork. This fork is the lowest frequency fork that can be manufactured, and though somewhat large and unwieldy, the penetrating qualities of the very low frequency have been shown to be very beneficial, with people reporting feeling very relaxed after the tone has been applied to the body. The fork is imprinted with the letters *Y H V H,* which is Hebrew for "I Am Who I Am," the name of Creator. Through Hebrew Gematria, a system of assigning a numerical value to a word or phrase, the value of the name YHVH (Yod, Hey, Vav, Hey) is $10 + 5 + 6 + 5 = 26$ (the tetragrammatron, one of the names of God in the Hebrew Bible). Hence I have nicknamed it "the G-d Fork."

In the years since I have also incorporated a weighted 111-Hz fork (111 is the negative space between many of the Solfeggio frequencies), and more recently I had a 62.64-Hz fork custom made for me. I chose this frequency because I thought it was the eighth harmonic of the Schumann resonance, or 7.83 Hz × 8 (more on this in later chapters), but I later learned that because of the curve of Earth and the atmosphere, the higher harmonics of this frequency are not necessarily perfect multiplications of the fundamental. Regardless, this particular frequency fork has shown itself to be very powerful and useful.

The application of weighted forks appears to open space up within the body. Just as the 5- to 7-Hz frequencies employed in the conventional medicine practice of lithotripsy create space between the molecules of a kidney stone or gallstone, breaking them into smaller pieces, the sound current travels through the different mediums of the body, inducing an opening and relaxation of clenched areas. This allows blood, lymph, and electricity to flow with greater efficiency through the area, speeding the body's process of healing and balancing itself.

2020 update: In the years that followed the first publication of this book, I went on to create additional weighted forks: 54.81 Hz and 93.96 Hz (called "the Sonic Slider"), which are also based on the Schumann resonance, as well as the Fibonacci Pair, 89 Hz and 144 Hz. I no longer use the 111-Hz fork or the 26-Hz forks.

INCORPORATING A CRYSTAL INTERMEDIARY

One day a client came to a session with a crystal that she told me was a Lemurian seed crystal, a quartz crystal with a typically frosted appearance and subtle striations that look as though they've been lasered on the crystal. These crystals were first found in Brazil in 1999, lying separately in a bed of sand, unattached to clusters, which is the normal way quartz points are found. She asked if we could use it during the session. I was skeptical and not even sure what to do with it. I ended up resting it right on her body over the second chakra when I was almost done balancing it. I immediately noticed that the tone came in clearer, brighter, and faster; it seemed to add efficiency to the process (after all my years of working in a busy restaurant, anything that added efficiency was a winner to me). Intrigued, I asked if I could borrow it, and proceeded to incorporate it into each session that week.

I reluctantly gave the crystal back to her at week's end and then did a session without it, where it became quite clear to me that I needed one of my own. Fortunately, I didn't have to look very far. There was a rock and bead shop right in my hometown where they happened to have an assortment, and in short order I had a Lemurian seed crystal of my own. I was now an official crystal-packing New Age healer!

For about six months, I used it as I had initially, by placing it directly on whatever chakra I was working on toward the end of the process. But then one day I figured out another way to use it. I was working on a young woman who was lying face-down on the table. She was wearing a spaghetti-strap tank top, and so it was easy to see that her shoulder and upper back muscles were hard, flat, and rigid. She had been complaining about all the tension in them. Up until this point I had been placing the handles of my forks on trigger points, but in this moment the mail slot opened and a note dropped in. It said, "Run the sound from the tuning fork through your crystal into her body." So I did—I placed the sharp end of the crystal on a trigger point and the handle on the flat end, and my jaw dropped as I watched the muscles in her back immediately plump up, like a baby's bottom. I repeated the process on the other side of her spine, with the same outcome. "What did you just do?" she exclaimed. "I have no idea," I replied. She stood up and rotated her shoulders. "They're so relaxed! Wow!"

I was so astounded by this dramatic outcome that I immediately began trying to figure out what had happened and why. I learned two things that seemed to explain this episode. One is that quartz crystals both amplify and pulse whatever kind of current is run through them. This is the reason why quartz is used as a timekeeper—it sets up a rhythmic and predictable pulse when an electrical current runs through it. So the crystal had translated the sound current into amplified pulses.

The other thing that seemed to be a factor was the possible stimulation of nitric oxide (NO) production. Before this experience, a client had brought me a flier he had picked up at a health fair that claimed that tuning forks have been shown to increase the production of nitric oxide in the body. It said that NO is a gas that causes muscles to relax and blood vessels to dilate. Listening to certain types of music and other practices also stimulate this response.

Putting two and two together, it seemed to me that the amplified pulse of sound had hyperstimulated NO production, leading to this dramatic and immediate relaxation effect in this region of my client's body. From that time on I began to regularly use the Lemurian seed crystal in this way. In hindsight, however, I have come to see that this person was an outlier—while the process always is relaxing to people, I have never had anyone since then have such a dramatic response to it. The unique combination of her dramatic response and the fact that because of the way she was dressed I could see her response made her an ideal candidate for the mail slot to choose that moment to introduce the idea to me.

BEGINNING TEACHING

In 2010 I began to teach the method. I was reluctant to do so until I had completed my master's degree, but I had a group of clients who were unwilling to wait that long, and they coerced me into starting a class with them. My pilot group had ten people in it, and we set out to see if the method I had developed could be taught. I found that everyone was able to master the click, drag, and drop process fairly quickly. People were, and are, surprised to discover that they can hear and/or feel the resistance in the field when they encounter pockets of stuck energy and then can move it.

It's a curious thing to teach adults to locate and manipulate something that is both subtle and invisible, but our organization has trained well over two thousand people at this point and we have yet to encounter anyone who cannot do this. Older folks, over sixty, have a harder time hearing, but they still always manage to sense when they have come across something significant. My students began reporting outcomes like the ones I had grown accustomed to seeing: diminished pain, settled emotions, experiences of greater clarity and peace, and the like.

As a result of my teaching the method, for the first time I was able to have the experience of receiving this work myself, which was very instructive. I was able to tell what it felt like to have energy move around, and also to experience the benefits of it. Some of the outcomes of my receiving the work were greater emotional stability and clarity, a cessation of the clicking in my shoulders that happened whenever I raised my arms up, less of a tendency to have midback pain, and the complete disappearance of seven very stubborn plantar warts on the sole of my left foot (I've had other people report disappearing plantar warts as well).

And teaching the method led me to become even more concerned about the questions I was having all along: What the heck is it that we are moving around? What laws of physics are governing this process? Am I making all of this up? What other kind of research has been done regarding the human energy field and therapeutic sound? I had been unable to turn up anything in the esoteric literature that answered any of these questions to my satisfaction, and so I used my master's degree as an opportunity to do academic research on the subject.

4

USING SOUND
THERAPEUTICALLY

From Ultrasound to Music
Therapy—How Sound Is Used
in Alternative and Conventional
Medicines

*Every illness is a musical problem—the healing, a
musical solution . . .*

NOVALIS, *THE ENCYCLOPEDIA* (1772–1801)

While getting my undergraduate and graduate degrees, I was given the opportunity to write several research papers on therapeutic audible sound and was extremely surprised to find a complete dearth of information in the academic literature about its application and practice. Searches yielded information on the use of audible sound for tinnitus and autism, and little else. There was research on infrasonic sound, as used in the practice of lithotripsy (using 5- to 7-Hz pulses to break up kidney stones); and there was research on ultrasonic sound as used in physical therapy to stimulate blood flow to areas; but there was virtually nothing on the use of single tones of audible frequencies.

This made me aware of a curious fact: the use of inaudible sound was considered conventional, and the use of audible sound was considered alternative. Using tuning forks as I had since 1996, I had encountered quite a lot of skepticism. People seemed to have no problem accepting that a 7-Hz frequency directed at their kidneys could relieve their kidney stones, but could not accept that a 174-Hz frequency directed at their head could relieve their migraines.

There was no logic to this, but I found over and over again that most mainstream-oriented people had an immediate and predictable ideological rejection of the notion that audible sound frequencies could produce a beneficial therapeutic outcome. And it was easy to see why: there had been virtually no related American published research, and we are culturally programmed to reject anything that hasn't been validated by the scientific method.

Needless to say, this made doing research challenging. I had to look to other areas of research to find uncontroversial, accepted parallels. The logical first step was to look at music research. Music therapy has been a relatively accepted mainstream practice since after World War II, when it was used to treat veterans suffering from posttraumatic stress disorder, or PTSD. Quite a lot of research has been conducted on music, especially in the last decade, when fMRIs (functioning magnetic resonance imaging, a system to image brain activity related to a specific task or sensory process) have made it possible to see what's happening in the brain in real time.

While I did find some interesting correlations, especially regarding the concepts of resonance and entrainment (discussed below), after some consideration I realized that the sound work that I was practicing was much more targeted and specific than music therapy. Additionally, the concept of an interface with the energy field surrounding the body was a significant part of the work I was doing, and this played no role at all in music therapy.

Thus, because there was so little to draw from in the academic realms as I was putting together my research, I was forced to look to studies and examples from outside of academia, which in the end seemed appropriate because sound is used in both alternative and conventional medicines.

CONVENTIONAL VS. ALTERNATIVE
APPROACHES TO SOUND IN MEDICINE

My research revealed an interesting phenomenon that I had not previously considered with regard to the different perceptions and applications of sound in conventional and alternative medicines: conventional medicine employs sound frequencies in the ultrasonic and infrasonic ranges, while alternative medicine largely employs frequencies in the audible range. While the practice of using these ultrasonic and infrasonic frequencies is well documented and widely employed in conventional medicine, there has been very little attention given to the use of audible frequencies. The two perspectives break down along distinct lines, with just a little overlap. I will first discuss the uses of sound as found in conventional medicine.

Ultrasound

Perhaps the best-known and most widely employed use of sound in conventional medicine is in the use of ultrasound. Most people are familiar with its use as a diagnostic technology, as in the use of sonograms for viewing a fetus in utero; the sound waves bounce off the bones and fluid and return the information to a transducer, which translates it into a visual image of the unborn infant. Medical sonography is also used diagnostically to discover pathologies within the body.

Ultrasound is also used therapeutically. Ultrasound therapy has been shown to cause an increase in tissue relaxation, local blood flow, and scar-tissue breakdown. The effect of the increase in local blood flow can be used to help reduce local swelling and chronic inflammation, reduce pain, and, according to some studies, promote bone-fracture healing.[1] It is regularly employed by physical therapists and chiropractors. However, despite over sixty years of clinical use, there are few studies that definitively verify the efficacy of therapeutic ultrasound. One of the reasons for this is the challenge presented by trying to make this a double-blind process, whereby both the investigator and the participant are blind to (unaware of) the nature of the treatment the participant is receiving.

This issue makes studies on the effectiveness of sound challenging due to the aforementioned numerous channels of conductivity. Some more recent studies have been more conclusive; one shows a 44 percent reduction in trigger-point sensitivity after just one five-minute application of high-intensity ultrasound.[2]

Ultrasound can also be used to evoke phonophoresis, a noninvasive way of enhancing the absorption of analgesics and anti-inflammatory agents to tissues below the skin by means of ultrasonic waves.[3] Incidentally, we have found that tuning forks can also be used this way; when the handle of weighted forks is applied to different stones or crystals, essential oils, or flower essences, it seems to have the effect of driving the vibration of the medium deeper into the body.

Newer Applications of Ultrasound

Ultrasound is also being used as a noninvasive surgery technique. Magnetic resonance–guided focused ultrasound surgery (MRgFUS) is a process that uses highly focused ultrasonic frequencies to destroy unwanted growths such as fibroids and even tumors by rapidly heating them. The magnetic resonance provides a precise guidance system to focus the sound beam on the specific area and then raises the temperature there to the point where the structural integrity of the growth is destroyed. Although this treatment has been in use since 1994 and has been used on fibroids, breast tumors, prostate tumors, and more, showing highly successful results, it has been slow to catch on. An important difference between high-intensity focused ultrasound surgery and many other forms of focused energy, such as radiation therapy or radiosurgery, is that the passage of ultrasound energy through intervening tissue has no apparent cumulative negative effect on that tissue.[4]

Another sound application in conventional medicine is the practice of lithotripsy, a technology that breaks up stones in the kidneys, gallbladder, or liver with pulsed infrasonic sound waves in the range of 4 to 12 Hz; these smaller pieces of stone are in turn more easily passed by the body. This technology was developed in the early 1980s in Germany and has since become more widely used, but can bring on complications at the rate of 5 to 20 percent and can also result in a sensation akin to being punched in the kidney.

Last, a search of *sound therapy* in a medical database will bring up mostly articles about the use of tinnitus retraining therapy (TRT) to treat tinnitus, the phenomena of a constant ringing or roaring in the ears. While apparently no cure for this has been determined, TRT is an ongoing process that uses sound generators to help sufferers retrain their relationship with the issue so that it no longer bothers them as much, a process that can take upward of two years to be truly effective.

SOUND MEDICINE USED IN BOTH ALTERNATIVE AND CONVENTIONAL SETTINGS

Music therapy, vibroacoustic therapy, and the Tomatis Method are three techniques that are used both conventionally and alternatively. All three fall into the category of sound therapy.

Music Therapy

As mentioned earlier, music has been used clinically in the United States since World War II, when it was used to treat veterans suffering from PTSD. Since then it has become more widely employed and is now used in hospitals, nursing homes, institutions, and other rehabilitative settings. Music therapists work to help clients improve their level of functioning and quality of life by using music experiences such as singing, songwriting, listening to and discussing music, and moving to music, to achieve measurable treatment goals and objectives.

Music therapy has been shown to be particularly effective with some of the more challenged members of the population, especially those with Alzheimer's disease and dementia, autistic spectral disorders, stroke victims, and even prisoners. A study on a group of women in prison in Israel who all participated in a choir showed that group members "experienced a sense of community and togetherness as a result of the exercise."[5] Alzheimer's patients demonstrate less agitation and confusion when engaged in group or individual music exercises, as opposed to being left alone in front of a TV.[6] Autistic children are able to be more expressive and engaged when involved in musical activities.[7]

Music is also gaining more acceptance in the medical field, being used during surgery and postoperatively, and especially in the practice of music thanatology, which combines music (often harp music) with end-of-life care. According to Daniel Levitin, professor at McGill University and author of *This Is Your Brain on Music,* "Music initiates brainstem responses that, in turn, regulate heart rate, pulse, blood pressure, body temperature, skin conductance, and muscle tension, partly via noradrenergic neurons that regulate cholinergic and dopaminergic neurotransmission."[8] It is also being used to help people manage pain, anxiety, stress, and a surprisingly wide range of other issues.

Studies have shown the method of music therapy that works most effectively uses the principles of resonance and entrainment. Entrainment music therapy is described as "any stimuli that matches or models the current mood state of the individual and then moves the person in the direction of a more positive or pleasant mood state."[9] For example, if a person is initially agitated, the music selected will match that agitation initially (i.e., resonate with), and then move slowly into a melodic piece that can lead to anxiety reduction (i.e., entrain to). This technique has been used successfully in the reduction of both pain and anxiety.

It is my observation that tuning forks may work on the same premise and that this is potentially central to their therapeutic efficacy. Initially, they resonate with whatever dissonance may be present, gradually entraining, through the inherent coherence and order of the produced tone, the dissonance of the body into a more harmonious expression. For example, if someone is experiencing pain in a particular area, when the fork is initially held over that area it will sound either sharp or full of static. After a few moments, however, the noise can resolve, or settle down, and the fork will sound more harmonious. People often report a simultaneous reduction in discomfort. This principle is one of the reasons why acoustic sound therapies are different (and potentially more effective in some cases) than synthesized sound therapies; the "living" quality of the acoustic tone allows for this reflective resonance and entrainment to occur.

Vibroacoustic Sound Therapy and the Tomatis Method

Vibroacoustic Sound Therapy (VST) incorporates both music therapy and sound frequencies. VST is the transduction of both sound and music through specially designed beds, tables, or chairs, with speakers arranged in such a way that the sound currents travel directly through the body. Lower frequency waves, in the range of 30 to 100 Hz, are generally used, and sessions can last from ten to forty-five minutes. This technology originated in Sweden in the 1970s and is now used worldwide in settings ranging from hospitals to spas. Many studies have been conducted on this technology and have demonstrated that it is beneficial in addressing a wide range of ailments, from pain and anxiety reduction to reducing problem behavior in autistic adults and children. One study found that negative stereotypical behavior was reduced upward of 40 percent in autistic adults.[10]

VST can be used with just music, pulsed sound waves and music, and in some technologies, combined with visual light stimulation. Most studies have determined that VST is most beneficial when pulsed sound is combined with music, and nearly all studies have shown that it brings improvement in a wide range of disorders.[11]

The Tomatis Method, and a somewhat similar technology called Auditory Integrative Training, are other sound therapy techniques that have undergone some rigorous studies. While these therapies are fundamentally different, both involve listening to specially created music through headphones for the purpose of retraining the auditory system and creating symptomatic improvement for issues such as autism, learning disorders, hearing disorders, ADHD, and more. The treatment of autism has been the most studied with these techniques, as they are generally effective at reducing the sound sensitivity so commonly found with this disorder, resulting in improved interaction with the person's environment.[12]

SOUND IN ALTERNATIVE MEDICINE

The use of sound in alternative medicine is much broader and deeper than what is found in conventional medicine. For the purpose of this part of the discussion it is important to distinguish between sound healing and sound therapy. *Sound healing* refers to the more general field of therapeutic sound use, including singing, drumming, rattling, toning, etc., whereas *sound therapy* refers to methods that are more clinical and structured. In alternative medicine, sound therapy is a subgroup of sound healing.

The Human Voice

Conscious and intentional use of the human voice in chanting, singing, and toning has been around for millennia, often within a religious or devotional context. Many studies have been done to determine what exactly happens when we chant or sing or tone, whether alone or in groups. When experienced meditators engage in chanting meditation, neurological imaging has shown changes in blood flow to the brain, in addition to other biological markers of increased well-being.[13] One study demonstrated a positive emotional effect and immune competence confirmed by the increased presence of secretory immunoglobulin A in saliva swabs after a choir rehearsal and an even more marked increase after a performance.[14]

The process of toning, which has gained some popularity in recent years, is a sort of informal chanting wherein the person simply intones extended vowel sounds, which in turn supposedly helps release energy blockages from the body. Chanting is said to have a similar result of facilitating the flow of energy through the body.

Tuning Forks, Gongs, and Singing Bowls

Acoustic instruments such as tuning forks, gongs, and crystal or Tibetan bowls are widely used in sound healing. One of the best-known tuning fork practices, called Acutonics, is a system developed by an acupuncturist in which vibrating weighted tuning forks are used on acupuncture points. Its effectiveness is based on the same premise as acupuncture—that stimulation of these particular areas unblocks stuck or stagnant energy, improving energy flow throughout the body and supporting the body in healing itself. Acutonics is being employed in some hospitals and nursing homes.

Unweighted tuning forks are also used on and around the body. Because this is my particular area of expertise, I have attempted to find studies that demonstrate the effectiveness of this technique to address pain, anxiety, and some of the other issues my clients report frequently, but I have been unable to turn up a single scientific paper supporting this use. John Beaulieu, one of the authors of an article titled "Sound Therapy Induced Relaxation: Down Regulating Stress Processes and Pathologies," states on his website, www.biosonics.com, that he discovered that tuning forks spike the body's production of nitric oxide (NO)—yet tuning forks are not referenced in the above-mentioned article he coauthored. Nevertheless, Beaulieu and his fellow authors speculate that the physiological reason why music and sound therapy induce relaxation is because of the relaxing properties of NO, which appears to be released in the presence of certain music and sounds. According to Beaulieu, NO is not only an immune-, vascular-, and neural-signaling molecule, it is also "antibacterial, antiviral and it down-regulates endothelial and immunocyte activation and adherence, thus performing vital physiological activities, including vasodilation."[15]

Crystal and Tibetan bowls are another common feature of sound healing. These are struck or rubbed to produce pure, penetrating tones not very different from those produced by tuning forks. Metal bowls have been used in Tibet for centuries as an aid to meditation, while crystal bowls are a relatively recent development; both are used similarly. Dr. Mitchell Gaynor, an oncologist and author of *The Healing Power of Sound,* began integrating music, vocalization, breathing, sound, and meditation techniques in his work with patients in 1991, after first being exposed to a Tibetan bowl through one of his patients. He observed many beneficial outcomes as a result of this integration, such as reduced stress, greater tolerance of chemotherapy, as well as a sense of community within the groups that met regularly for sound meditation.

Other Sound Technologies

Binaural beats are created when two tones are de-tuned from each other by a small amount. The resulting third oscillation, which is the difference between the two frequencies, automatically entrains the brain into different brain-wave frequencies. For example, if 315 Hz is played into the right ear and 325 Hz played into the left ear, the brain becomes entrained toward the beat frequency of 10 Hz, which is in the Alpha brain-wave range, the range associated with relaxation. Binaural beats are embedded in music or simply as repeated tones and listened to through headphones.

Various studies suggest that the therapeutic application of binaural-beat technology can be beneficial for anxiety, mood improvement, behavior disorders in developmentally disabled children, and stress reduction in patients with addictions and focus and attention problems.[16]

BioAcoustic Biology, a technique developed by sound pioneer Sharry Edwards, is the use of human-voice analysis to provide a representation of a person's state of health. This technology reads the frequencies present in a person's voice and determines which important frequencies are missing. Once appropriate sound formulas are ascertained, they are programmed into something called a *square 2 tone box,* a portable analog frequency generator that allows a person to listen privately through headphones or a subwoofer. According to Edwards's website, BioAcoustic therapy has had success with a broad range of issues, but several specific areas stand out for their success rates: sports injuries and structural problems, pain management, nutritional evaluation, and tissue regeneration.

I was unable to find any published studies on this technology. All of the studies that are available appear to have been done by Sound Health, Sharry Edwards's own research organization. However, the second edition of *Alternative Medicine: The Definitive Guide* includes

BioAcoustics as a recommended alternative therapy, one of only four sound therapies listed. Furthermore, in 2009 Edwards received the Scientist of the Year award from the International Association of New Science.

Another notable entry in the energetic medicine field is Cymatherapy (aka Cymatic Therapy), a frequency-generating technology developed in the 1960s by Dr. Peter Guy Manners, a British osteopath who devised his method after many years of research into harmonic frequencies. The Cyma-1000 unit used in this technology emits over five hundred different frequencies. Some fifty years of research behind this method have determined which frequencies and combinations of frequencies treat which ailments; it then uses an applicator to deliver precise combinations of frequencies associated with healthy tissue and organ systems. The theory is that these sound waves help to normalize imbalances and synchronize the cell's frequency back to its natural healthy state of vibrational resonance.

This technology is used and accepted in the United Kingdom (where it is referred to as "advanced medicine," rather than alternative medicine) but not so much in the United States, where it is registered with the FDA as an "acoustic massager." I was unable to find any peer-reviewed studies on the Cyma-1000 (or on any of the other frequency generators currently available, such as the Rife machine, Medisonix, and others), although composer and sound healing pioneer Dr. Gary Robert Buchanan, author of *SONA: Healing with Wave Front BIOresonance,* has been involved in research with this technology for the last thirty-eight years, at the Cosolargy Institute in Reno, Nevada. He claims to have come up with sonic solutions for a variety of issues, including a recent advance in eliminating cataracts without the need for surgery.

I recently saw a YouTube video interview with Cymatherapy's founder, Dr. Peter Guy Manners, which took place in the United States in the early 1980s. He was convinced back then that he was introducing a technology that was going to revolutionize medicine in this country; now, almost thirty years later, it seems Dr. Manners's predictions are coming to pass, and this type of sound medicine is finally beginning to gain acceptance.

Dr. Manners was not the first person to work with audible frequencies therapeutically and to develop a large body of work related to it. Royal Raymond Rife was another researcher who developed a technology, beginning in the 1930s, that used both audible and inaudible frequencies, both diagnostically and therapeutically. His Rife machine is based on the premise that each pathological organism has a threshold at which a particular frequency shatters it, like a wine glass shattered by an opera singer. By increasing the intensity of the naturally resonating frequencies of these microbes, Rife created structural stress that caused them to distort and then disintegrate, without harming any of the surrounding tissues. He called this frequency the "mortal oscillatory rate." Rife spent many thousands of hours in exhaustive research developing a specific process that involved directing these frequencies through a plasma tube, which was filled with helium gas that turned into a plasma with the introduction of an electric current, and applied to the area of pathology in the patient. Rife reported many amazing cures, including cancer, through this process. Unfortunately, his work was destroyed, his lab burned, and his reputation ruined, allegedly by Morris Fishbein, the head of the American Medical Association at that time.[17]

The aforementioned technologies represent the sum total of my academic research into sound and frequency technologies and practices. It's important to note that there are many more technologies and practices beyond what I have shared here, but I limited my research so as to find as much peer-reviewed information as I could. Sound and frequency healing is a field that is growing tremendously at the moment, but there is currently no journal of sound healing practices. And because, as I mentioned earlier, studies on sound healing cannot be double- or even single-blinded, approaching research from a traditional perspective is, for all intents and purposes, nearly impossible.

Aside from the information about receptor antennas, or primary cilium, on cell membranes and their tuning fork–like nature, along with the fact that successful music therapy intervention employs the principles of resonance and entrainment just like tuning forks appear to, very few of my questions had been answered up to this point in my research. The dearth of relevant information on this subject led me to believe I was quite alone, on the fringe of a frontier where there were few peers and where there had been little scientific work undertaken that could answer my questions. I was particularly concerned with understanding the physical composition of the energy and information that I was encountering in the body's energy field, as it was my sense that there was actual "stuff" there that I was manipulating. While esoteric literature discusses the spiritual properties of the human energy field, it neglects to mention whether this field is composed of free electrons, biophotons, magnetic fields, or other such scientifically described phenomenon.

Nevertheless, the next two turns in my journey supplied me with unexpected and welcome answers to my persistent questions.

5

WIDENING MY UNDERSTANDING OF PLASMA AND AETHER

How the Electric Universe Theory and Schumann Resonance Relate to Healing

We are star stuff contemplating the stars.

CARL SAGAN

The first turn occurred one night at the family dinner table, when my son Quinn, who was twelve at the time, announced, "Did you know there was a fourth state of matter called plasma?" At the time I had to say that I did not in fact know there was a state of matter called plasma. I was familiar with solids, liquids, and gases, but somehow the fact that there was something called *plasma* had eluded me.

In that same conversation we had been discussing the vacuum nature of space. I must confess that my limited science education (I had avoided both physics and chemistry in high school and college) had left me with a rather rudimentary understanding of such things, but I had a vague recollection of having read once somewhere that space is not, in fact, a vacuum of empty nothingness like I had been taught, but that it is actually filled with something.

After dinner I did an internet search of "space is not a vacuum" and was only mildly surprised to discover that space, in fact, appears to be filled with none other than plasma. That began my journey down the plasma rabbit hole. I spent the next five months researching plasma every spare moment I could, and the information I uncovered caused me to completely reframe my cosmological outlook. I became so enamored of what I was learning that my husband said to me at one point, "You don't love me—you love plasma!"

PLASMA

Before we begin a discussion about plasma, the fourth state of matter, it is important that we understand exactly what plasma is. Usually when I start to talk to people about plasma I have to say, "It's not blood plasma, it's the other plasma," and then I am usually met with a blank stare. The fact of the matter is that the majority of people have no idea what plasma is, which is a curious fact when one considers that plasma comprises as much as 99.99 percent of our universe.

The reason why most people do not know about plasma is because they are not educated about it in school. Like me, most people are only taught about solids, liquids, and gases. And while education has changed a bit in recent years, most NASA press releases—the way by which many of us seem to learn about space phenomena—refer to the stuff that is technically plasma as "hot gas" most of the time. It's a shame, really, that more people don't know about plasma, because plasma is actually quite a fascinating and even exciting concept.

So, what then is it? Here are a few definitions:

- *Plasma* (physical chemistry): a fourth state of matter distinct from solids or liquids or gases and present in stars and fusion reactors. A gas becomes a plasma when it is heated until the atoms lose all their electrons, leaving a highly electrified collection of nuclei and free electrons. (WordNet Search)
- *Plasma* consists of a gas heated to sufficiently high temperatures

such that the atoms ionize. The properties of the gas are controlled by electromagnetic forces among constituent ions and electrons, which results in a different type of behavior. Plasma is often considered the fourth state of matter (besides solids, liquids, and gases). Most of the matter in the universe is in the plasma state. (Solar Physics Glossary)

So, then, plasma is a gas that conducts electrical current. It is different from regular gas in that the electrons have been separated from their nuclei, leaving a "soup" of negative electrons and positive ions. Generally, it is referred to as the fourth state of matter, although many sources point out that it should technically be called the first state of matter, as it is what the other three states arise from (or technically, condense from).

What are some examples of plasma? Well, our sun for one, as well as all the stars in the sky, and all the space between those stars as well. Here on Earth we see plasma in the form of lightning strikes and the northern lights, and daily in the form of fluorescent lightbulbs, neon signs, and plasma TVs. Who knew that plasma was so abundant and ubiquitous?

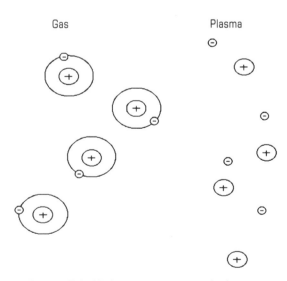

Figure 5.1. Hydrogen gas turned plasma

Another place we see plasma is in the fascinating pictures of nebulas that the Hubble telescope is sending back from space (although, again, these are usually described as "hot gas"). Plasma is also used in business, industry, and health care. Most people have heard of a plasma cutter or an arc welder. These technologies make use of hot plasma. Nonthermal or cold plasma is used as a sterilizing agent in the food industry and also in the medical profession, as it has been discovered that it can sterilize hospital and food production equipment quickly and inexpensively. It can also be used to speed wound healing. Plasma is actually quite a growth industry at the moment, full of promising developments.

Let's take a look at some of the properties of plasma.

Properties of Plasma

Many researchers who have studied plasma have remarked on its "almost lifelike" qualities. Plasma spontaneously forms filaments, cells, and sheaths. These helical, twisting filaments in space are called *Birkeland currents,* named after Norwegian researcher Kristian Birkeland. He demonstrated that electric currents flow along filaments shaped by current-induced magnetic fields. As plasma filaments come together by means of long-range attraction, they rotate around one another. This creates a short-range repulsive magnetic force that holds the filaments apart so that they are insulated from one another and thus maintain their identity. They rotate faster and faster as they draw together, forming a helical structure. These twisting helical structures carry electrical currents over vast distances, connecting stars and interstellar space, somewhat like electrical wires.

Plasma forms cells of different voltages, temperatures, densities, and chemical properties, and separates these cells by means of what is called a *double layer* (DL) *sheath*. This double layer consists of a positively charged layer separated from a negative layer by a small, electrically charged space. This sheath provides the cell with protection against its environment. For example, the sun's heliosphere is bounded by a DL sheath. When a foreign object is inserted into plasma, the plasma will immediately form a sheath around it. It is this tendency to isolate any intruders that may have led American chemist and physicist Irving Langmuir, who coined the name *plasma* in 1927, to name it as such after *blood plasma,* which has the same tendency. This quality makes plasma difficult to measure because it will isolate any recording devices.

Plasma is recognized as having three modes of operation:

1. Dark current mode, or low current. This mode does not usually emit light. Ionospheres (plasma sheaths) of planets and interstellar space are examples.
2. Normal glow mode, a stronger electric current. In this mode the entire plasma glows. Neon signs, auroras, comet tails, and the sun's corona are examples.
3. Arc mode, a very strong current. This mode forms very bright twisting filaments. Electric welders, lightning, sparks, and the sun's photosphere are all examples. In general, the stronger the current, the brighter the plasma.

Plasma research has been conducted over the last century by a variety of researchers, and more recently important work has been done on plasma by American physicist Anthony Peratt, who created some interesting computer simulations that show how electrical Birkeland currents give rise to galaxies. He, along with author-scientists Wallace Thornhill and Donald Scott, are key players in plasma research today. In fact, these scientists are proponents of a whole new way of looking at the cosmos, called the Electric Universe theory, which states that electricity, not gravity, is the key defining force in the universe.

THE ELECTRIC UNIVERSE THEORY

*From the smallest particle to the largest galactic
formation, a web of electrical circuitry connects and
unifies all of nature, organizing galaxies, energizing stars,*

giving birth to planets and, on our own world, controlling
weather and animating biological organisms. There are
no isolated islands in an electric universe.

DAVID TALBOTT AND WAL THORNHILL,
THUNDERBOLTS OF THE GODS

The most profound concept I have ever come across in any of the research I have done in my entire life is the emerging cosmological theory called the Electric Universe (EU) theory, which is an outgrowth of plasma cosmology. Put simply, EU says that electricity, not gravity, is the dominant force in space. Up until this point, astrophysicists insisted that charge separation cannot happen in space, and they therefore dismissed the electric force as an impossibility. However, information sent to us by space probes and the Hubble and other telescopes has demonstrated the truth of this charge separation. It would now seem that it can no longer be denied that electricity is a force—perhaps *the* defining force—in space.

EU is a radical departure from our current cosmological model. In EU there is no need for black holes, dark energy, dark matter, or other strange things we cannot see. What many people do not realize about these phenomena is that they are all mathematical constructs, not observed realities. These imagined entities have been conjured up to explain how the insufficient gravity in galaxies can account for them hanging together. But according to EU, all observable phenomena in space can be easily described and predicted because plasma is scalable—meaning the plasma created in a lab behaves in much the same way as the plasma we see in space.

Gravity has been perceived as the dominant force in the universe for over three hundred years; the entire scientific revolution was built on this cosmology. It should come as no surprise that the academic world is not taking too kindly to these revelations about EU, and that the theory is shunned in many academic circles. Despite academia's skepticism, it has been said that EU is a revelation on par with the work of Copernicus and Galileo or the quantum physicists at the early part of the last century. Just as Bohm, Bohr, Einstein, and others created a revolution in thinking by redefining our perception of the micro—the quantum world—Peratt, Thornhill, and Scott are creating a revolution in thinking by redefining our perception of the macro, the universe. It is paradigm-shattering in a very powerful way because it is a retelling of our cosmological story.

The cosmological story is the most important story in a culture. It forms the backdrop that every other story is written against. All human dramas play out on a stage, with the cosmos as the overarching, defining pattern. Our current cosmology goes something like this: 13.7 billion Earth years ago, there was a point that was "infinitely hot and infinitely dense," which exploded and has been expanding ever since. It will keep on doing so until, according to the second law of thermodynamics, it will all spread out, dissipate, and end. Galaxies are held together by gravity, by black holes in the middle that "devour" light, and by mysterious dark energy pushing them together from the outside. Everything else is mysterious dark matter.

In this dark and mysterious universe, life is random, chaotic, and pointless. Everything is machinelike and separate from everything else. You and I really can't understand any of it because our cosmologists define most of what is going on in space—in terms of how old it is and how fast it is expanding—with complex mathematical formulas. Many reports from NASA speak of scientists being puzzled or confused about the phenomena they are witnessing in space. It's a hostile, dangerous, and confusing territory.

But that isn't how EU sees it at all. In EU everything hangs together; everything makes sense. The Electric Universe theory both explains and consistently predicts space phenomenon based on the predictable behavior of electromagnetic plasma. One of the things I say in my lectures is that the best self-help book I ever read isn't even a self-help book: it's *The Electric Sky,* by Donald Scott, which clearly and concisely lays out EU theory in such a way that anyone can understand it. Here was what I had been looking for all along without even realizing it—a cosmology of connectivity, of light, instead of separation and darkness. I suddenly saw, and felt, how I was connected to the rest of the universe, and this revelation of connection was nothing short of a love affair. My husband was right—I had fallen in love with plasma.

Our sun, instead of being an isolated thermonuclear furnace of hydrogen gas fusing into helium gas (a self-sufficient individual, burning itself out), is an electric dynamo, powered by galactic Birkeland currents and connected through this web of electricity to every other electrically powered star in the universe. This explains why stars and galaxies form in strings along these massive intergalactic power wires, not so very different from Christmas lights on a string. It is the large-scale filamentary structure predicted in the 1960s by Hannes Alfvén, Swedish electrical engineer, plasma physicist, and recipient of the 1970 Nobel Prize in physics, which has been verified by galactic observation since the '80s. It is also an image that is often shown next to artists' renditions of the neural web of circuitry of our brains.

The solar wind, which really isn't a wind at all but an electrical current, delivers a flow of electrical energy to Earth, which is also an electrically charged body. Earth has a plasma DL sheath that serves as a buffer for this flow of electromagnetic energy; this is called the *magnetosphere*. When the electric discharge from the sun is high, we see the auroras form at the poles. The electricity discharges its buildup in lightning strikes and also travels across and under the surface of the Earth and the oceans in *telluric currents*. These natural, earthbound electrical currents have been mapped, and these maps are owned and used by oil and gas companies, presumably to find deposits. Apparently they were also used to power the early telegraph system in the United States.

When I first learned about telluric currents, I couldn't help but wonder if they were the same thing as dragon lines, the filamentary Earth currents of chi described in Chinese feng shui, or the ley lines of Neolithic Europe, which I understand are "tamed" dragon lines, straightened and used by our ancestors in much the same way we can straighten a river and turn it into a canal—same phenomenon, different name. I started to wonder if diffuse plasma and chi were the same thing, and if the human energy field was just a sort of a plasma bubble with a double-layer sheath at the outer boundary.

BIOPLASMA

Following this line of inquiry, I was able to come across other information that likened the human energy field to plasma, calling it *bioplasma,* or the fifth state of matter. The following paragraph appears in numerous sites on the internet (but I was unable to find any references to the original work of Inyushin):

> Since the 1950s, Dr. Victor Inyushin at Kazakh University in Russia has also done extensive research in HEF (Human Energy Field). He suggests the existence of a bioplasmic energy field composed of ions, free protons, and free electrons. He suggests that the bioplasmic energy field is a fifth state of matter. (The four states are solids, liquids, gases, and plasma.) Inyushin's work shows that the bioplasmic particles are constantly renewed by chemical processes in the cells and are in constant motion. There is a balance of positive and negative particles within the bioplasma that is relatively stable. A severe shift in this balance causes a change in the health of the patients or organism.[1]

Barbara Brennan, a former NASA physicist and a world-renowned energy healer, also refers to the human energy field as a *bioplasma;* she sees physical trauma as "frozen" or stuck energy within this bioplasmic medium.[2] Ampère's circuital law states that wherever there is an electric current, there is a magnetic field. According to research by Rollin McCraty et. al.:

> Compared to the electromagnetic field produced by the brain, the electoral component of the heart's field is about 60 times greater in amplitude, and permeates every cell in the body. The magnetic com-

ponent is approximately 5000 times stronger than the brain's field and can be detected several feet away from the body with sensitive magnetometers.[3]

The SQUID, or superconducting quantum interference device, is an extremely sensitive magnetometer capable of measuring the biomagnetic field produced by a single heartbeat, muscle twitch, or pattern of neural activity in the brain. This instrument is now being used at universities and medical research centers around the world in order to better understand the role of the biomagnetic fields in the diagnosis and treatment of medical conditions.

Here is what the HeartMath Institute has to say about the electromagnetic field of the heart:

> The electrical energy produced by the heart radiates outside the body into space. The heart's field is not static. It changes, depending on what we are feeling. For example, when we are feeling emotions like anger or frustration, the frequencies in the field become chaotic and disordered. On the other hand when we are experiencing emotions like compassion, care, appreciation or love, the frequencies in the field become more ordered and coherent. In a sense, through the electromagnetic field created by the heart, we are literally broadcasting our emotions like radio waves.[4]

This notion is slightly different from what is generally associated with the human energy field, which shows bodies of different densities and properties, as seen in figure 5.2 (on page 94). The rings are referred to as *koshas,* or *sheaths,* again stemming from the Vedic tradition. Both perspectives describe the field as toroidal (doughnut-shaped). The torus (or toroid) is a shape that repeats throughout nature as in the toroidal nature of the plasmaspheres of Earth, the sun, and a photon.

When one considers that the human body carries an electrical charge and also has a north and south pole, the larger toroidal

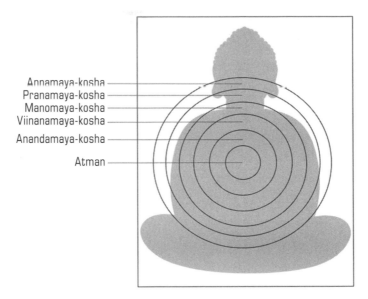

Annamaya-kosha
Pranamaya-kosha
Manomaya-kosha
Viinanamaya-kosha
Anandamaya-kosha
Atman

Figure 5.2. The koshas, or sheaths, of the aura

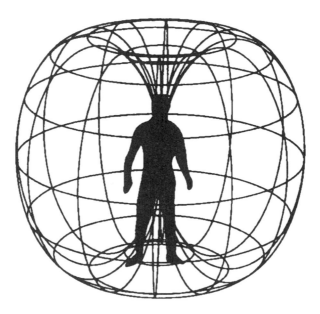

Figure 5.3. Hypothetical toroidal field of the human body

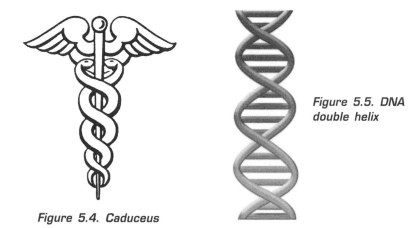

Figure 5.5. DNA double helix

Figure 5.4. Caduceus

representation in figure 5.3 seems plausible. Remember that plasma is described as forming twisting filaments, cells, and sheaths. The DL sheaths are formed at the outer boundaries of the plasma field and have a higher electrical charge than the ambient plasma within the boundary defined by the sheath. It would make sense that since the human body also has an electromagnetic charge, it would repeat this pattern, since life expresses itself in fractals*—in short, "as above so below."

When plasma in arc mode (like lightning or a plasma welder) travels across distances in space, it forms the twisting Birkeland currents mentioned earlier, which spiral around one another. This vortex or spiraling action expresses itself in life-forms on many different levels; it therefore makes sense that it is also present in the subtle body.

Vedic literature describes the two serpentine channels that begin at the base of the spine and spiral up to the crown of the head, creating chakras, or vortexes of energy, at each crossing point. These images bring to mind two other common images, the caduceus (figure 5.4) and the DNA double helix (figure 5.5).

The caduceus is an esoteric symbol that various texts describe as originating in ancient Egypt. It features two snakes, representing the two etheric channels that comprise kundalini energy running up

*The term *fractal* was coined by mathematician Benoit Mandelbrot in 1975 to refer to the nongeometric repeating patterns observable throughout nature.

through the body, connecting the lower physical and the upper spiritual realms of the body. The ida is the left, female channel, or yin energy, and the pingala is the right, male channel, or yang energy. The central channel or staff is the shushumna, which runs along the spinal column. When the mind is quiet, the shushumna becomes active, uniting the inner self with the cosmos. The wings of the caduceus represent the air element associated with the upper, spiritual self, the exploration of which comes with the balance of the channels, and the staff itself is made of metal, which represents the element of earth.

Other sources describe the caduceus as arising from later Greek mythology and associated with the god Hermes (or Mercury, as rendered by the Romans). In this form the caduceus has been recognized as a symbol of the marketplace.[5] Thus it would seem that the Greeks and Romans took an esoteric image that originally expressed the primal aspects of the masculine and feminine energies as related to the upper spiritual energies and applied it to commerce, as opposed to one's inner elemental experience. The idea of the marketplace taking the place of the cosmos and our own inner riches is true particularly in our modern world. Perhaps ironically, this esoteric symbol has been adopted by our mainstream Western medical system and appears as a logo for many health-care practitioners and companies, including the American Medical Association.

Figure 5.5 (page 95) is a depiction of the helical structure of DNA. From the micro to the macro, we see the movement of energy forming into these complementary, helical structures of negative and positive, feminine and masculine, yin and yang. So it would appear that the flowing electrical plasma in space is very closely related to the flow of energies within our own body.

We have been conditioned to think of ourselves as chemical and mechanical beings, but we are also extremely electrical. Most people think of the nervous system when they think of electricity in the body, but it has been determined that collagen, the connective tissue that is present everywhere in our bodies, is also a conductor, that our blood carries a charge, that our bones conduct electricity, that our heart is an electrically driven oscillator, and that our brain waves are electrical frequencies.

THE SCHUMANN RESONANCE

Curiously, human brain waves can function in the same wavelength as a frequency that is generated in the cavity between Earth and its ionosphere by all the lightning strikes going on all over the world in any given moment, which averages approximately two hundred storms producing fifty strikes per second. This frequency, a 7.83-Hz standing wave and its higher harmonics, which are present as a continual electromagnetic pulse in our environment, is called the Schumann resonance. It is sometimes referred to as the "Earth's heartbeat." This ambient frequency is received by our pineal gland, which is composed of about 30 percent magnetite, a type of iron oxide with natural magnetic properties, and appears to be important for governing a variety of functions, including melatonin production and the regulation of the endocrine (hormonal) system. When astronauts first started going up into space outside of Earth's atmosphere, they reported getting "space sickness" from pineal malfunctioning, which seemed to be a consequence of not being exposed to this continual background governing frequency. When Schumann resonance generators were placed aboard spacecraft, this issue was mitigated.

Interestingly 7.83 Hz is also a brainwave frequency associated with meditative and creative states and is often recorded in shamans and healers. Brainwave states are generally divided into four categories: delta (0–4 Hz), associated with deep sleep, renewal, and healing; theta (4–7 Hz), associated with insight, intuition, and awareness; alpha (7–13 Hz) associated with calm, relaxed alertness; and beta (13–40 Hz), associated with nervousness, irritability, anger, and the like. The brainwave activity of most modern humans is in the beta range. It would appear that when our brainwaves are in sync with the Schumann resonance (in the alpha state), we are in an optimum frame of mind.

We tend to think of lightning as a cloud-to-ground phenomenon;

however, it has been discovered that it is actually an ionosphere-to-ground phenomenon. Various electrical phenomenon, called *elves,* *jets,* and *sprites,* have been observed and photographed between the tops of clouds and the upper atmosphere while lightning strikes are happening below cloud level. Since the ionosphere is in constant electrical contact with the sun through the solar wind, and the sun is in constant electrical contact with the rest of space through the connective Birkeland currents, we are, through the electrical activity in our own brains and bodies, literally resonating with the rest of the electrical universe, especially when we are tuned in to the 7- to 8-Hz wavelength. This is also the frequency that has been measured coming out of the hands of chi gong healers when doing healing sessions—meaning they are truly channeling universal electromagnetic energy.

CREATING A NEW COSMOLOGY

We are electromagnetic beings, bathed in an electromagnetically connected reality—all really is one in this very simple way—but we have been disconnected from this awareness and trapped in a paradigm that only teaches us about solids, liquids, and gases. In this old model we live in Newton's gravity-driven, billiard-ball universe, spinning meaninglessly through a cold and disconnected vacuum of space. Despite the comment by 1918 Nobel Prize–winning physicist Max Planck, that "we have now discovered that there is no such thing as matter, it is all just different rates of vibration designed by an unseen intelligence," we still live as though we are in the world of the discrete, disconnected particle, the self-sufficient individual, in which mind and body, human being and nature are separate, discrete entities.

I propose that the reason why the current reigning paradigm hasn't really shifted out of this illusion of separation is because we have only part of the story—the micro part. Quantum theory tells us that everything is connected at the scale of the very small. But Electric Universe theory describes a vibrating, connected macro, and in doing so it changes the cosmological story of the last three hundred years. When our cosmology changes, everything else changes, because everything refers back to cosmology.

People yearn for a sense of connection. This sense of connection, of an underlying current of interrelationship, is essentially what we know as spirituality, oneness. The cosmology of the scientific revolution has been one of separation, of spiritlessness. EU shows us how we are all connected via plasma.

But there is yet another, deeper connecting layer: aether.

AETHER

According to the general theory of relativity, space is endowed with physical qualities; in this sense, therefore, there exists an aether. According to the general theory of relativity, space without aether is unthinkable.

ALBERT EINSTEIN

Let's look at the dictionary definition of the word *aether:*

1. Any of a class of organic compounds in which two hydrocarbon groups are linked by an oxygen atom
2. A volatile, highly flammable liquid, $C_2H_5OC_2H_5$, derived from the distillation of ethyl alcohol with sulfuric acid and used as a reagent and solvent. It was formerly used as an anesthetic. Also called *diethyl ether, ethyl ether*
3. The regions of space beyond Earth's atmosphere; the heavens
4. The element believed in ancient and medieval civilizations to fill all space above the sphere of the moon and comprised of the stars and planets
5. *Physics:* An all-pervading, infinitely elastic, massless medium formerly postulated as the medium of propagation of electromagnetic waves

So, we are not talking about definitions 1 and 2, but rather what is alluded to in definitions 3 through 5. Note that in definition 5, this all-pervasive, infinitely elastic, massless medium was formerly postulated as being the medium of propagation of electromagnetic waves. So, from this we may deduce that aether is an all-pervasive medium that is everywhere in the universe all at once.

Aether was once understood as being the medium through which starlight propagated, but this meaning was removed from science in the early 1900s and replaced with the vacuum theory, presumably in support of Einstein's theory of relativity. The textbook explanation for why the concept of aether was removed from science refers to an experiment conducted in the late 1800s called the Michaelson-Morley experiment, whose null outcome supposedly demonstrated that aether, as it had previously been conceived, did not really exist. The story about the people and the experiments concerning this subject is a fascinating one, but I won't go into it in detail here. Suffice it to say that the general supposition, when it comes to Einstein and aether, was that he at first believed it did not exist, but by 1922 had come to the opposite conclusion—that there had to be an aetheric medium in space.[6]

Despite the fact that Einstein recanted his earlier assertion that aether did not exist, by then the concept had fallen out of fashion, and it has remained in disfavor up through our present time. But the need of late to have some kind of explanation for this subtle, all-pervasive energy field has reasserted itself, and so over the last century this medium has been reintroduced with a variety of new names: *the zero-point field, the source field, the quantum potential, the field,* and even *the Higgs field,* whose definition, "an invisible energy field that exists throughout the universe," sounds an awful lot like the definition of aether.

THE SELF-AWARE UNIVERSE

Now, if you think back to my earlier description of subtle energy in the first chapter, you will see that it appears that when we talk about aether, we are talking about the same thing. But wasn't I just wondering a few pages back whether plasma and chi are the same thing? Now am I suggesting that aether and chi are the same thing? Good question—I'll do my best to explain it as I have come to understand it.

Because of the structure of our language, we tend to think of stuff in our environment as "things," but if you think back to what Max Planck said about everything being vibrations of different frequencies, "things" are really more like processes. Notably, the Hopi and other languages contain no nouns, but rather refer to everything as if it were a *process that is happening* instead of a *thing that is*.

Matter and energy in our environment are constantly transforming. Frequency states shift along a continuum, a spectrum in which there are no real divisions. Sunlight gets absorbed by trees and they become bigger trees; water evaporates and becomes water vapor; stars explode and become star dust. There are different key thresholds where one state of matter becomes another—for example, the liquid of water becoming the solid of ice. But ultimately there is simply a single spectrum of electromagnetic frequencies that vary, from the very high and fast to the very low and slow.

In the continuum of all matter, we have aether, the highest and finest and most basic state of matter, which spins itself through torsion spirals into concentrations called *plasma*. This in turn condenses into gases, liquids, and solids, ultimately forming the stuff we see around us. It would appear that subtle energy exists in a great number of degrees of density or texture, ranging from very subtle to more coarse or tangible. From what I can tell, everything from the finest aether to a diffuse plasma can be called *subtle energy*. And all of it is potentially consciousness. Here's why: To hang together as a cohesive unit, which it is, the universe must have some degree of self-awareness—it must be conscious of itself, and it must be instantaneously conscious, with no lag time in the signaling, meaning the information transfer in this medium must be faster than the speed of light. And this medium, the aetheric medium that exists everywhere throughout the universe, serves as the medium through which the universe is self-aware.

This concept of the self-aware universe can also be seen in the concept we call gravity—all of the universe must have instantaneous awareness of itself everywhere at once, or else how could it remain in relationship with the degree of order that it has?

I was thinking one morning about how universal self-awareness is a property of aether, which is present everywhere all at once, and that I had read that gravity was also described as having these same traits, when I suddenly wondered how gravity and aether were related. I did an internet search of "gravity is a property of aether" and found that there are people who espouse the theory that rather than being a force that pulls us down, gravity is in fact a force that pushes us down: it is the force of the all-pervasive yet subtle aetheric field that is pushing from all around into the center of Earth.

This made me think about neutrinos and how they are described as massless high-frequency particles that very weakly interact with matter, and how they push in on the surface of Earth from all directions. Could what science calls *neutrinos* be the same thing as aether, I wondered? So I searched that too. And I found that Wal Thornhill, one of the leading proponents of the Electric Universe theory, says exactly that.

Now remember, I am not saying that any of this is definitely so. I'm not an expert; I'm a student, a person asking questions. I'm simply sharing with you some of the answers I have come up with and showing you how they *could* fit together. I absolutely encourage you to do your own investigation and form your own opinions about the material I am presenting here.

Okay, let's keep looking at the properties ascribed to aether, because this is important. Remember that there are many different names for this particular phenomenon, but since *aether* was the original name, it is the one I choose to use.

Aether is described as operating holographically, meaning the whole is present in every part. It is aether's holographic nature that allows for instantaneous communication without regard for time or distance—meaning that aether is the medium of consciousness, the carrier wave of it, so to speak. As the nonlocal interconnective medium that unifies us all in real time, aether is the missing link in so-called paranormal phenomena such as remote viewing, distance healing, synchronicities (i.e., meaningful coincidences), and telepathy.

According to physicist Paul LaViolette, author of *Secrets of Antigravity Propulsion,* the hidden "aether physics" explains how UFOs are able to navigate in the rapid zig-zag and up-and-down fashion that has routinely been witnessed. LaViolette, who has done extensive research into these subjects, asserts that the awareness of aether has been intentionally suppressed for a number of reasons, "national security" being one of these.

The scientist Nikola Tesla (1856–1943), who invented AC power and many other things besides, figured out a way to harness and transmit the energy of aether. We do not learn about Tesla and all his amazing contributions to science in our educational system. It is not conspiracy theory to take note of this, but rather an awareness of simple economics: Tesla wanted to transmit free energy to everyone, and his financier, seeing the implications of this, pulled the plug on his advanced technologies. He was then subsequently written out of our official history, while aether was written out of official science.

Aether is also described as moving in torsions or spirals, and as such it is called the *torsion field* or *torsion waves.* We see how nature repeatedly coalesces in these spiral patterns; from galaxies to snail shells to weather patterns, the proportions of the Phi spiral repeat on every level of creation. The Phi spiral and corresponding Golden Mean rectangle (1:1.618) are proportions that repeat themselves fractally throughout nature (see figure 5.6 on page 104, the golden ratio).

The spiral is not the only pattern characteristic of aether. The five Platonic solids (see figure 5.7 on page 105) are also part of the underlying geometry of creation that arises in aether. These solids were first described by Plato as being the only forms that fit perfectly within a sphere, connected by identically shaped surfaces, edge lengths, and angles—an identical view in all directions. The Greeks taught that

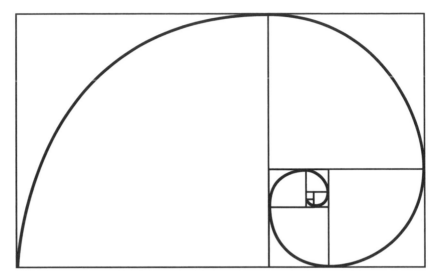

Figure 5.6. Phi spiral and Golden Mean rectangle

these five solids were the core patterns of physical creation. Four of the solids were seen as the archetypal patterns behind the four elements—earth, air, fire, and water, what we know as the four states of matter. The fifth was held to be the pattern behind the life force itself—the Greeks' aether. This fifth solid, the dodecahedron, was in fact kept a closely guarded secret in the Greek school of Pythagoras, and even Plato spoke little of it. They feared that this pattern could cause tremendous destruction if misused. (Looking at that shape makes me think of the Pentagon!)

These patterns, like the spiral, also appear throughout nature, especially at the atomic level in chemistry. And the shape that is not shown, the sphere within which all of these forms can nest, is yet another one of the fundamental forms of aether. When you combine a sphere with a spiral, you get the torus, another fundamental pattern within aether.

In the esoteric tradition it is said that the human body has an aetheric template, a subtle-energy matrix in vortex/torus form that channels and stabilizes the aetheric energies, making them more dense and

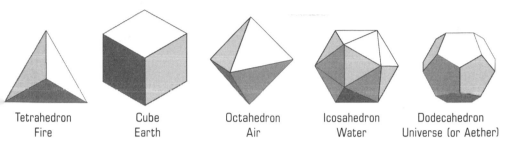

| Tetrahedron | Cube | Octahedron | Icosahedron | Dodecahedron |
| Fire | Earth | Air | Water | Universe (or Aether) |

Figure 5.7. Platonic solids and states of matter

charged, and eventually responsible for creating the physical body. The aetheric template comes first, followed by the body. It is the human mind that creates the shape or structure of the torus for the length of a lifetime. When the mind withdraws at death, the toroidal construct, the underlying pattern that gives rise to order, ceases to exist, and the physical body falls apart.

Although the torus shape of the aura has a boundary—the double-layer sheath of plasma cosmology—it sits in the universal aetheric field, which is unlimited, or infinite. This is also the reason why we are all connected, at all times, with everything else in the universe. So if we insert aether and plasma into our cosmological framework, we suddenly have a dimension beyond the material world that we are accustomed to.

The presence of aether, with its holographic, everywhere-at-once-ness, is a simple and plausible explanation for things like telepathy, distance healing, distance viewing, and all the other paranormal practices that are dismissed as impossible by the aetherless conventional paradigm (no need to call it what Einstein termed it, "spooky action at a distance"). Our consciousness, being ultimately nonlocal and part of this holographic soup, is free to wander at will, to connect instantaneously to other minds, even at great distances. Especially for people whose brainwaves are in the Schumann range, synchronistic events become the norm, as these persons allow themselves to be guided by Thoreau's subtle magnetism.

With regard to healing, in aetheric or spiritually based practices, one can directly alter this aetheric body and create physical changes in the physical body. That is because if you can manipulate the aether and the plasma, you can manipulate the physical. The so-called biofield therapies work precisely on this premise, as we shall soon discover.

6

DISCOVERING THE BIOFIELD IN SCIENCE

The Concept of the Biofield and the Biofield Tuning Biofield Model

The existence of a "bio-field" or "bio-energetic field" directly contradicts principles of physics, chemistry, and biology.

VICTOR STENGER

Authority in science exists to be questioned, since heresy is the spring from which new ideas flow.

JOHN POLYANI

After reading about plasma and bioplasma, I felt that I was onto something. However, aside from Barbara Brennan and the elusive Russian and Chinese research, the only other researcher whom I could find espousing a similar idea was Jay Alfred, author of *Our Invisible Bodies*. In this book Alfred outlines the logic involved in the concept of "higher harmonic electromagnetic energy bodies," but then he goes on to use the explanation to describe ghosts and life after death, both off-topic concepts to my research. Additionally, Alfred holds no degrees. I was having a very hard time finding American scientists who were researching the human energy field (the phrase I was typing into academic databases), until the next key turn in my research road, when I came across the word *biofield* in the book *The Energy Healing Experiments,* by Gary Schwartz, a professor of psychology, medicine, neurology, psychiatry, and surgery at the University of Arizona and the director of its Laboratory for Advances in Consciousness and Health.

According to Schwartz, the term *biofield* was chosen by a 1994 panel of National Institute of Health (NIH) scientists to describe the field of energy and information that surrounds the human body. Suddenly, my searches in PubMed and Medline began to bear fruit, and I became aware of a small but earnest group of American scientists working to describe the composition and mechanics of this field. No longer alone and out on the fringe, I found myself awash in the rich and useful contributions of those who had come before me in this same quest to understand and define something that the mechanists of old-paradigm thinking had been exerting a strong effort to sweep under the rug. It turns out that the mechanists have been attempting to dismiss the other camp, called the vitalists, for quite some time, insisting that there is no such thing as the life force.

With this term, *life force,* we run into a 400-year-old problem (some sources cite it as a 2,500-year-old problem): the fundamental disagreement between the mechanists and the vitalists over the nature of life. In *Energy Medicine: The Scientific Basis,* James Oschman, Ph.D., a world authority on energy and complementary medicine, describes it this way: "Mechanists hold that life obeys the laws of chemistry and physics. Vitalists have historically held the belief that life will never be explained by normal physics or chemistry and that there is some form of mysterious 'life force' that is separate from the known laws of nature."[1]

This debate took center stage in 1784 with the drama that came to surround German physician Franz Anton Mesmer. Again, quoting Oschman: "In 1773, Franz Anton Mesmer began using magnets for healing. His patients frequently noticed 'unusual currents' coursing through their bodies prior to the onset of a 'healing crisis' that led to a cure. Soon Mesmer discovered that he could produce the same phenomena without the magnets, simply by passing his hands above the patient's body."[2]

Mesmer claimed that he detected a magnetic fluid that surrounded the body, and he formulated a theory closely akin to Chinese medicine. Mesmer had come to see health as the free circulation of life energy through multiple channels in the body and illness as blockages in this circulation. It was his observation that dislodging these blockages to restore flow could potentially create a healing crisis, followed by restored health. When the body is unable to unblock itself, the intervention of a conductor of what he called *animal magnetism* was both required and effective in assisting this process.

What is particularly interesting to me regarding Mesmer is that I too have had the same experience or feeling sense—that there is indeed a sort of magnetic fluid surrounding and interpenetrating the body, and that blockages in this field are representations of blockages within the body. Where energy does not flow, pathologies arise. Unblocking the energy in the field can lead to a resolution of the issue in the body. The coherent tones produced by activated tuning forks appear to act as a conductor of animal magnetism, in that they have the capacity to unblock the flow of the life force, or free up "frozen" bioplasma.*

Unfortunately, a panel of scientists that included the late, great Benjamin Franklin decided in 1784 that Mesmer's "magnetic fluid" and "animal magnetism" were figments of his imagination. He was barred from practicing medicine and went on to live the rest of his life in exile and obscurity. And science has maintained this particular stance ever since, with the mechanists trumping the vitalists. Yet despite the dismissal of Mesmer, there have been a number of scientists in recent times who have been pushing forward with scientific inquiry, regardless of the prevailing paradigm of mechanism.

---

*In plasma physics, the study of the movement of plasma is called *magnetohydrodynamics,* implying the presence of a magnetic fluid.

PIONEERING BIOFIELD RESEARCHERS

One of the first Americans to do extensive academic research on the electromagnetic fields surrounding matter was Harold Saxton Burr, a professor of anatomy at Yale Medical School from 1929 to 1973. From 1932 to 1956, Burr conducted extensive work exploring these energy fields, which he termed *L-fields*.[3] During this time he was going against the current of mainstream biology and medicine, which was geared toward the mechanistic and pharmaceutical model.

Despite the fact that his peers considered the concept of life fields to be complete nonsense, Burr was convinced that his L-field was the blueprint of living matter. According to him, if a disturbed energy field could be detected and returned to normal, pathology could be prevented from arising. While not accepted in his time, his work became the basis of a later researcher, Robert Becker (1923–2008), an orthopedic surgeon by profession. Becker was the author of the classic book *The Body Electric: Electromagnetism and the Foundation of Life,* and one of his many contributions was to demonstrate that acupuncture points are special regions of higher electrical conductivity than the tissue surrounding them.[4] Becker also believed that the electromagnetic fields in and around the body are primary for giving rise to and organizing the physical body.

More recently, Rupert Sheldrake has put forward the concept of morphic resonance and morphic fields. Sheldrake has been a controversial figure in contemporary science because of his determinedly vitalist perspective (he is one of the fellows I mentioned earlier who was censored by TED). He describes morphic fields in the FAQ of his website in this way:

The hypothesis of formative causation states that the forms of self-organizing systems are shaped by morphic fields. Morphic fields organize atoms, molecules, crystals, organelles, cells, tissues, organs, organisms, societies, ecosystems, planetary systems, solar systems, galaxies. In other words, they organize systems at all levels of complexity, and are the basis for the wholeness that we observe in nature, which is more than the sum of the parts. . . . Morphic fields also contain an inherent memory given by the process of morphic resonance, whereby each kind of thing has a collective memory. For example, crystals of a given kind are influenced by all past crystals of that kind, date palms by past date palms, giraffes by past giraffes, etc. In the human realm this is similar to Jung's theory of the collective unconscious.[5]

Sheldrake's argument that morphic fields give rise to the order, structure, and function of organisms points to a holistic, nonreductionist view of nature. He notes that "the shift from a mechanistic to holistic paradigm of nature has been happening in stages for several decades, but mainstream science is still committed to a mechanistic and reductionist view of nature."[6]

This perspective underscores the primary difference between the viewpoints of mechanists and those of vitalists. The mechanistic view is that any biological fields in the body are a consequence of the presence of physiological activity, whereas vitalists argue that the physiological activity is a consequence of the electromagnetic and other subtle energies present. This argument is summarized in the statements that we are either a "spiritual being having a physical experience," or a "physical being having a spiritual experience." My personal opinion is that we are both, as each gives rise to the other in a dynamic and continual exchange. Light is, after all, both a particle and a wave from the human perspective.

Certainly much of the biofield research of the last few decades, as Sheldrake notes, underscores the validity of the vitalist perspective. In her seminal 2002 paper, "The Biofield Hypothesis: Its Biophysical Basis and Role in Medicine," Beverly Rubik, Ph.D., describes the biofield as a complex, weak, electromagnetic (EM) field that utilizes EM "bioinformation" for self-regulation. This is an underlying light grid of speed-of-light (essentially instantaneous) communication that underlies the much slower chemical processes that it gives rise to. This is what accounts for the rapid and holistic effects of some complementary and alternative medicine (CAM) therapies that purport to work within this field.

Rubik points out that CAM practices such as acupuncture, homeopathy, and bioelectric medicine, as well as biofield therapies like Reiki, therapeutic touch, and healing touch (Biofield Tuning falls in this category as well) all work within the underlying EM field, but that these therapies remain outside the mainstream because there is no agreed-on scientific foundation to describe how and why they work. She describes how physics had to be changed in the early part of the twentieth century to accept the observation that light behaves as both a particle and a wave, and says that particle-wave duality needs to be considered because life consists of both complex biomolecular structures and dynamic waves of information. Looking at life from the molecular/chemical/mechanical perspective provides a scientific basis for allopathic medicine, while looking at it from an energetic/biofield perspective offers a scientific foundation for many CAM modalities.

Seen from this perspective, the human body is not only composed of physical, mechanical, and chemical components, but also has an oscillating electromagnetic aspect, with each cell, organ, and system contributing to a complex standing wave of many different frequencies that change over time, not unlike a symphony.

Because the body is a collection of dynamic frequencies, the introduction of outside frequencies such as that produced by a tuning fork, a homeopathic remedy, or even a drug, could potentially change, strengthen, or destabilize the biofield. This frequency modulation, working as it does with the underlying blueprint, can produce a biological response. This description is a possible explanation for how and why audible sound frequencies interface with the biofield as they do, producing beneficial therapeutic outcomes. The following statement by Rubik supports this idea:

Many natural frequencies are emitted by the brain and heart, and externally applied fields at these same frequencies can cause entrainment and physiological, psychologic [sic], and behavioral changes. Siskin and Walker (1995) have reviewed the healing effects of specific frequency windows, and some of them are as follows: 2 Hz, nerve regeneration; 10 Hz, ligament healing; 15, 20, and 72 Hz, stimulation of capillary formation and fibroblast proliferation. This suggests that EM bioinformation is fundamental to regulation of biologic [sic] function, and that it is encoded in the biofield. Thus, the natural oscillators in living systems themselves emit EM bioinformation regulating biologic function. In other words, cells and tissues may be "whispering" EM signals to one another and "listening" for relevant signals from their surroundings.[7]

Rubik proposes that the biofield hypothesis "provides the rudiments of a scientific foundation for the energy medicine modalities of acupuncture, homeopathy, bioelectromagnetic therapies, and biofield therapies."[8] The first stage in the modus operandi of these modalities is predicted to be an interaction with the organism's biofield, and the result is an effect on homeodynamics, the organizing intelligence of the body that always seeks to promote healing and maintain order and balance.

OTHER BIO-ENERGY RESEARCH

Dr. William Tiller, professor emeritus of materials science and engineering at Stanford University and a pioneer in the field of subtle-energy research, has taken this idea even further. While Dr. Tiller's work lies beyond the scope of this book, it is noteworthy that he and his colleagues at Stanford developed a subtle-energy detector, an ultrasensitive Geiger counter–type device with which they have demonstrated the existence of an energy field that is not in the known electromagnetic spectrum. Dr. Tiller was able to demonstrate with this device, as well as with a variety of other devices and methods, that this subtle energy responds to human intention and focus.[9]

Another American scientist, the late Dr. Valerie Hunt, research scientist, author, lecturer, and professor emeritus of physiological science at UCLA, also studied the human biofield for decades and made many contributions to this field of research: "Postulating that human bio-energy fields oscillate at significantly higher frequencies than EKG or EEG machines were designed to measure, Dr. Hunt developed a high-frequency instrument which records the bioelectrical energy that emanates from the body's surface. She proved that energy radiating from the body's atoms give frequencies 1,000 times faster than any other known electrical activity of the body."[10]

Dr. Hunt also conducted research using an electromagnetically shielded "mu" room and found that when electromagnetism was removed from the room, people "went to pieces," having emotional breakdowns for no particular internal reasons. When ambient electromagnetic energy was restored to the room, participants found themselves feeling fine again.[11] This implies that the presence of EM fields is necessary for an organism to maintain a sense of coherence and "togetherness."*

BIOPHOTONS

While Rubik, Tiller, Hunt, and other scientists discuss electromagnetic waves and frequencies, German biophysicist and researcher Fritz-Albert Popp describes the same phenomenon using a different term: *biophotons.* "In modern quantum theory, light occurs in small packets or particles of energy called photons. In living processes, certain specific types of photons are emitted and received primarily by the DNA, as well as a few large biomolecules. They serve as a function of com-

---

*I have come across several sources that claim that the magnetic field of Earth has declined 80 to 90 percent in the past four thousand years. When one considers this in relation to Dr. Hunt's study, it makes sense that we are seeing a steady rise in mental illness and a collective sense that the world is falling apart. It also makes sense that our ancestors were probably able to sense telluric currents (i.e., dragon lines) with much greater awareness because the currents were both a lot stronger and there was a lot less noise and EM interference than we have today.

munications, stimulation of biochemical reactions, and coordination within the body."[12] In other words, biophotons are quanta of coherent light that are thought to be emitted and absorbed by the DNA present in cells. Discovered by Popp in the 1970s, biophotons appear to create a holographic, coherent electromagnetic field throughout the body that uses EM frequencies for instantaneous communication throughout the systems.*

The science behind both biophotons and EM transmission describes a level of information below the level of chemical interactions. Sophisticated cameras have detected that the human body (indeed, all living organisms) emits these biophotons, with normal human emission from the skin between a few and a few hundred per square centimeter.[13] When an organism is under stress, however, it emits more biophotons. On the internet I found a picture of a soybean sprout that had been scored with a fine blade and photographed in a biophoton multiplier, an extremely sensitive device that can count the number of emitted biophotons. You can see quite clearly that the sprout is "leaking light" (i.e., creating greater biophoton emission, or leaking its life force) after it has been scored with a thin knife blade. Thus in the phrase "death by a thousand cuts," one is leaking not only blood, but perhaps one's vital organizing electromagnetic force as well.

The rapidly evolving field of biophoton research may be useful in bridging science and spirituality. Mystics have been telling us for millennia that we are beings of light; modern cosmologist and astrophysicist Carl Sagan has told us we are "star stuff." Now we can see precisely how the mechanism of coherent light may provide the energetic framework on which the physical body and its physiological processes take place.

British physicist Herbert Fröhlich (1905–1991) provided us with

---

*I had not thought about the similarities between the concepts of electromagnetic waves and biophotons until I started writing about them, but knowing that light appears as both a particle and a wave, it appears that regardless of the nomenclature, we are discussing the same thing. For those of us who are more particle inclined, the concept of a biophoton flying around the body may be easier to grasp than the concept of an EM wave.

greater insight into this mechanism. He believed that many biomolecules act as emitters and receivers of electromagnetic energy (as carried by biophotons) as well as vibrational energy (primary cilium, or the little tuning fork–like structures on the surface of cell membranes), and in doing so they provide the frequency required to allow specific reactions within the cells. Since most of the emitting and receiving is thought to happen through DNA molecules, biophotons act in a synchronizing fashion throughout the organism. This phase synchronization, which one could think of as all the parts of the body playing from the same sheet music, plays a crucial role in cell communication and coordination.

It may be that our DNA is a kind of antenna that receives and transmits information from our underlying aetheric/light-body template, and that our body maintains its coherence and organization from this inherent communication system based on information transmission of EM waves, and not on chemical signaling as is presently thought. Certainly the relatively slow process of chemical interactions cannot explain the incredibly rapid communication that is required for the actions of, say, an elite athlete.

What we have been discussing here, biophotons and electromagnetic signaling, defines the energy within the physical body itself. But what about the region beyond the physical body? Despite the popular notion that an electromagnetic field can only be detected a few millimeters off the body, the SQUID magnetometer has, by some accounts, been able to detect a faint magnetic field as much as twelve feet away from the human body.[14] I have certainly found this to be the case in my work with tuning forks, where I have been able to find information in a person's magnetic field six or more feet away from the surface of the skin. So what, then, is it exactly that constitutes the terrain that surrounds the body?

THE SUBTLE BODY

Claude Swanson, an MIT-educated physicist and author of the book *Life Force, The Scientific Basis,* states that biophotons remain within the body and that the terrain beyond is composed of what he calls *torsion waves* (also called *scalar waves* or *potentials*—possibly the same thing as aether). These non-Hertzian or longitudinal waves may emanate at right angles from the EM field produced by the body's electrical system, and they may be carriers of energy and information.[15] They appear to be of a much higher frequency and seem to underlie the traditional Maxwellian-Hertzian waves of the EM body (see the discussion of Maxwell in the section "What Is Energy," on pages 15–19). According to some mathematicians and scientists, the postulated longitudinal "standing waves" are conceived as "progenitors" or precursors of the transverse electromagnetic waves of Maxwellian physics, since it appears that interactions between pairs of these potential standing waves may generate the Maxwellian propagating waves of our more tangible world.[16] What this is saying, in short, is the same idea we visited earlier—that the higher, finer frequencies of aether come before plasma and actually give rise to it.

Subtle energy, like electromagnetism, comes in the form of the polarities of positive and negative and seems to exist as a sort of "higher harmonic" to electromagnetic energy, as it is present wherever electromagnetism is, yet is fundamentally different from electromagnetism in that it appears to obey different laws. For example, the research of German chemist, geologist, and naturalist Carl Ludwig von Reichenbach (1788–1869) into the nature of subtle or torsion energy, which he termed the *odic force,* or *od,* resulted in the following observations:

> When positive od is added to positive od, it results in a stronger concentration of positive od, with stronger effects. Likewise, when negative od is added to positive od, they tend to cancel. This additive nature of subtle energy leads to the use of the term "charge." Subtle energy charge is NOT electrical charge. Electrical charge exerts a very strong force, while subtle energy is usually much weaker. Electrical charge is conserved, which means that its quantity remains the same, it may flow elsewhere, but it does not simply

disappear. By contrast, subtle energy or od can decay over time and disappear.[17]

Another way to look at this subtle energy is through the Chinese concept of yin and yang. Yin represents the feminine or negative aspect, yang the masculine or positive aspect. In the previous chapter we mentioned the work of Russian scientist Victor Inyushin, who observed that the bioplasmic field around the body, which may be composed of free electrons, ions, and protons, demonstrates a balance of both positive and negative particles. When this becomes unbalanced, illness can ensue. Chinese medicine sees this as an imbalance in yin and yang energies and seeks to restore that balance. Below are some other representations of this polarity:

fire and water
electricity and magnetism
male and female
arriving and departing
dry and wet
white and black
red and blue
growth and decay
positive and negative
right-handed and left-handed
clockwise and counterclockwise
decreasing entropy and increasing entropy, or negative entropy and
    entropy

So, subtle energetic action appears to involve a torsion force, or spin, that travels in either a right-hand or left-hand direction. Depending on the direction of the spin, the energy takes on either a negative or a positive polarity. This spin is also attributed to the concepts of entropy and negative entropy, or *syntropy,* the term I prefer, coined in 1974 by Hungarian physiologist Albert Szent-Györgyi and proposed to replace the term *negative entropy.*

ENTROPY AND SYNTROPY

Entropy is defined as the tendency of a closed system to lose order over time. The Second Law of Thermodynamics states that entropy is inevitable in a closed system; the general common perception arising from this is that the Second Law predicts the ultimate dissolution of the universe. However, as Einstein notes, "The field is the only reality"—a statement that essentially means there are no closed systems in the universe, because everything, being ultimately waves, is without boundaries. The Russian astrophysicist Nikolai Kozyrev noted this:

> In the universe, however, there are no signs of the degradation which is described in the 2nd law of thermodynamics. Stars die and are born again. The Universe sparkles with inexhaustible variety. In it one finds no traces of an upcoming thermal and radioactive death. . . . Such systems, in a state of degradation, should prevail in the universe, and yet they are almost non-existent.[18]

Kozyrev concluded that when entropy increases in one place, it decreases in another. Rather than just disappearing, the force that gives rise to order in one place simply moves, or more precisely, radiates in torsion spirals to another place, where it will give rise to order there. So the overall entropy or level of order doesn't change, it just moves around. This idea is represented in figure 6.1 on page 120.

Depending on the direction of the spin, torsion is either syntropic or entropic, yin or yang. Now consider this quote by Buckminster Fuller: "The physical is inherently entropic, giving off energy in ever more disorderly ways. The metaphysical is antientropic, methodically marshaling energy. Life is antientropic."[19]

What begins to emerge is a curious picture of the Western mind being in denial of the antientropic, or syntropic, force. What Fuller is referring to when he says "the metaphysical" is the spiraling torsion force of subtle energy, the life force itself, the very same motion that gives rise to galaxies, planets, humans, snails, and flowers—this miraculous force

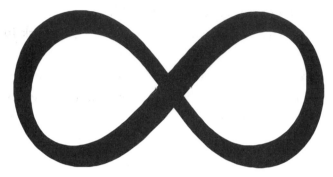

Figure 6.1. Infinite regeneration

that current science oddly insists on calling *negative entropy*. When this life force is present, in motion, it maintains order and structure and function. When it departs, entropy ensues.

The torsion field, or aether, is the ground state from which the visible universe arises. It is holographic, meaning all the information of the whole is available anywhere within it instantaneously. In this way it also acts as a record of everything that ever was: every thought, every feeling, every action. This concept is also referred to as the Akashic records.

Astrophysicist and sustainability pioneer Robert Gilman, founder and editor of Context Institute's journal *In Context: A Quarterly of Humane Sustainable Culture,** ties together the biological concept of morphogenetic fields—fields that literally "give birth to form"—and personal memories. He describes how the memories generated by our brains "are not locked in your brain, but are available throughout all space and all future time" through the process of morphogenetic resonance.[20] Gilman claims that not only is our biological form influenced by these fields, our behavior is as well, as shared memories influence behavior. Like Rupert Sheldrake, Gilman suggests that personal memories do not reside in the meat portion of our brain, but rather are vibratory patterns held in the zero-point field (torsion field, or aether) and can be accessed through our mind.

---

*Though no longer in print, many articles from this journal are available online.

So, how is all of this related to Biofield Tuning?

I encounter two fundamental phenomena in my work in the biofield, which I refer to as *energy* and *information*. The information is the record (memories) of everything that has occurred in a person's life, laid down on the torsion or aetheric level in what I perceive as standing waves. The energy is the charge associated with those memories.

While combing the area around the body with a vibrating tuning fork, I have the experience of encountering what appears to me to be charge, or electrical resistance, in the field. These pockets of charge appear to follow the tuning fork in a way that is reminiscent of iron filings following a magnet. Once returned to the spiral vortex of the chakra, the charge appears to be absorbed and "digested" by the body, implying that the charge prefers to be in the body rather than frozen or stuck in the field.

These charges appear to me to relate to trauma in a person's life. Periods of trauma, whether mental, physical, or emotional, often recede in time and space without ever being completely processed by the person (a process referred to in shamanism as *soul loss*). These memories seem to live on as charged incoherent oscillations within the biofield, exerting a nonbeneficial frequency pattern within the person's body and mind. Over time, they can create a breakdown in the order, structure, and function of the physical body (i.e., entropy). By locating, discharging, and neutralizing these dissonant frequency fields with tuning forks, and by returning the energy previously associated with them to the body, we are counterbalancing the entropy of the system, engaging in a syntropic process by manipulating the subtle energy or torsion field of the body. This is healing—the returning of order, structure, and function to the body.

But what is it, exactly, that I am moving? I call it *chi* when I describe it to clients, but I can't help but feel that there should be some kind of scientific word or descriptor for it. To my perception it behaves magnetically. Is it free electrons, free ions, or something exotic like magnetic monopoles? Could it simply be weak high-frequency biophotons? When I first came across the concept of biophotons, I wondered if I had found what I had been looking for. It made sense to me for a few reasons. It has been determined that an organism under stress emits more biophotons, which may be considered a "leaking of the life force." Does this lost energy simply dissipate in the collective aether? Could it somehow remain in our personal atmosphere as a kind of "soul fragment"? Could it be what I am combing up as I comb through the field with tuning forks?

It also seems to be connected to a quantum principle called Bose-Einstein condensation:

> When many photons of the same frequency and phase are present, they tend to pull other photons into the same state. Consequently, the high energy states tend to capture loose biophotons and get them to march in step together (like a laser). This is key to negentropy (syntropy). Instead of letting the photons spread out into many states, it pulls them into a few high energy states. In this way, it preserves order and reduces randomness or entropy. So Bose Condensation is one of the secrets of negentropy in living systems.[21]

This potentially explains several things, such as why the same patterns tend to repeat over and over again in our lives (for example, sadness over perceived abandonment)—because the biophotons in that part of our field keep drawing the experience to us (think Law of Attraction). It also explains how the tuning forks comb up these biophotons and return them to the center of the chakra, where they gain a more laser-like coherence. The increase in the coherence of EM emissions above a chakra after a Biofield Tuning session is evident in the way the sound produced by the tuning fork directly over the chakra is much louder and clearer after its field has been combed.*

---

*I have proposed the possibility of this charge being biophotonic to Claude Swanson—remember, in his model the biophotons exist only in or close to the body and the field is only torsion waves—but he does not agree that this is possible, contending that biophotons do not exist in the torsion field. I am hoping that future experiments with a biophoton multiplier might shed more light on my hypothesis.

Coming back to the idea of soul loss, or soul fragments, this apparent resolving of incoherent oscillations and integration of the charge associated with them back into the body is a process somewhat similar to shamanic soul retrieval.

Shamans say that during a traumatic experience, parts of the self get split off and left behind. The shaman enters into a trance state in order to locate and restore these lost pieces. When I first began employing the click, drag, and drop method within the field, I called it *sonic soul retrieval*. The outcome of locating, de-differentiating, neutralizing, and integrating these disturbances in the biofield can be immediate and profound, on all levels of functioning.

BIOFIELD TUNING BIOFIELD MODEL

According to neuroscientist and internationally recognized pharmacologist Candace Pert, author of *Molecules of Emotion,* "Your subconscious mind is really your body. Peptides are the biochemical correlate of emotion . . . They provide the body's most basic communication network . . . This means that emotional memory is stored throughout the body . . . and you can access emotional memory anywhere throughout the network."[22]

I would add that emotions are *electro*chemical events, with an aspect embedded in the body and the higher harmonic of that represented in the field. For example, by my own observation and also in Chinese medicine, the emotion of anger is stored in the liver. If someone has a lot of anger there will be a strong field of energy around the liver. When I manipulate the pattern of the field around the liver, discharging the energetic aspect of the electrochemical substance of anger, the physical body then potentially releases the chemicals. I have seen a number of situations where clients have experienced healing crises that include skin rashes, fevers, mucus, and flulike symptoms as a result of energetically discharging the liver.

This manipulation of the field may happen not only through the physics of entrainment of the dissonant frequencies, but also through the intention of the practitioner. The combined work of William Tiller, the Princeton University PEAR Lab (Princeton Engineering Anomalies Research, where consciousness-related physical phenomena were studied scientifically and in-depth from 1979 until 2007), and other scientists points to the fact that human intention influences reality through the manipulation of the electromagnetic and/or subtle-energy environments. This may be due to the fact that thoughts and emotions may be associated with electromagnetic events that also produce subtle energy. The subtle energy of the practitioner then interacts with the subtle energy of the client.

I have found that where I put my attention and intention is the level at which I am able to work successfully to effect a beneficial outcome. As I point out in chapter 7, in the region of the third chakra, or solar plexus, there are many different layers of information present: here we have the liver, gallbladder, stomach, spleen, pancreas, kidneys, and adrenals; here also is energetic information related to mother, father, the emotion of anger, and more. If I want to work on one specific thing— for example the adrenal rhythm—the mediating factor in this equation is my intention to work on this specific level. It is this ability to use my mind with this precision that seems to make the work so effective.

So, this brings up yet another challenging part of looking at all of this, and that is, what is the relationship between consciousness and subtle energy?

CONSCIOUSNESS AND SUBTLE ENERGY

Let's begin with some thoughts on the matter from leading minds in the field:

> *Neither science nor philosophy can even begin to explain*
> *how it is possible that mind, consciousness or spirit could*
> *influence matter or energy (subtle or electromagnetic).*
> *Nevertheless, the evidence is there, demanding explanation.*
> DAVID FEINSTEIN

As I understand the concept of qi (or ki, as it's called in Japanese), it's not just energy. It's really an intelligent energy, with consciousness attached to it. In other words, in Eastern philosophy, they never suffered a Cartesian split. So when they're thinking about an energy field around the body, it's not just physical electromagnetic or biophotonic fields, it's imbued with mind. It's something much more profound and not quite part of Western science.

BEVERLY RUBIK

Since we have consciousness, it is not unlikely, (according to the fractal nature of nature) that consciousness—a greater consciousness than ours of course, is everywhere.

MAUREEN LOCKHART

In order to fully understand and advance energy medicine (healing), science will have to accept the currently taboo possibility that pervasive intelligence (consciousness) exists throughout the universe.

GARY SCHWARTZ

The concept of a universal consciousness mediated by torsion waves propagating through the holographic aether or zero-point field (or quantum potential) can potentially explain the mechanics of how distance healing works. Just as I can place my awareness now in my left foot, now in my right hand, with no sense of that awareness having to travel in a linear way through my body, so I can place my awareness on a client a thousand miles away and use my subtle-energy field to influence it at a distance.

Numerous experiments have been conducted that demonstrate that qigong masters using a form of energy healing originating in China can create healing in one petri dish versus another over great distances, with great precision. Whether we place our awareness in a specific finger of the body or a specific petri dish far away, it is fundamentally the same action.*

Ultimately, science is coming to see what mystics have been saying for millennia—the universe is one unified field of varying frequencies, the arrangement of which determines the information present. The subtle field around the body is a field of potential, of energy, and information—in other words, a field of mind and consciousness.

That this field around the body even exists remains a subject of debate in modern medical science. Currently, the official stance of the American Medical Association and other related organizations, including all mainstream medical journals, is that the biofield does not exist. The reasons given for this are largely that it hasn't been sufficiently proven or adequately demonstrated, or, as noted by American particle physicist and author Victor Stenger, it "directly contradicts principles of physics, chemistry and biology."[23]

A good example of what constitutes the popular opinion on the biofield is the oft-cited study by Emily Rosa, the nine-year-old girl who in 1998 devised a science fair experiment to test the bioenergy sensitivity claims of practitioners of therapeutic touch, a practice that involves sensing and correcting disturbances in the biofield with the hands. Emily's science fair study showed that twenty-one therapeutic

---

*When seeking to understand the mechanics of distance healing, it is generally ruled out that EM energy plays a role, and for several reasons. Healing has been successfully conducted in EM-shielded rooms, and over great distances instantaneously, which would not account for the time involved for EM energy to travel. For this reason, torsion/aether is concluded to be the medium through which this energy travels. However, I have read that in EM-shielded rooms where there has been a biophoton multiplier, an extremely sensitive device that can count the number of biophotons being emitted by a life-form, "bursts of biophotons" have appeared while the distance healing is being conducted. This would imply to me that consciousness can "go under" in the aether in one spot and "pop out" in another instantly, without having to travel linearly to get there, in much the same way I can be conscious of and energize my right toe and then do the same with my left thumb, without that energy having to "travel."

touch practitioners were only able to sense when she held her hands up to theirs from behind a screen 44 percent of the time. Dr. Stephen Barrett of the organization Quackwatch (www.quackwatch.com) worked with Emily and her parents to write up the study and submit it to the *Journal of the American Medical Association,* where it was accepted and published, and subsequently picked up by the popular media.

Thus this study by a nine-year-old girl, coauthored by people who were extremely critical of complementary and alternative medicine, became unrefuted evidence that biofield therapies were groundless and unjustified.[24] However, Rosa and her coauthors failed to cite two previously published studies that used far more sophisticated designs, subjects, trials per subjects, and experimenters, all of which demonstrated that 66 percent of blindfolded college students could determine which of their hands was closest to the experimenter's hand. Studies conducted in 1995 and 1998 by Gary Schwartz and his colleagues demonstrated this and a variety of other basic mechanisms of biofield awareness, whereby they found approximately 15 percent of participants were 70 to 80 percent accurate in their perception of bioenergy. And many other rigorously controlled and replicated studies have also demonstrated the efficacy of other energy practices such as Reiki on such unbiased participants as rats and bacteria.[25]

Nevertheless, Schwartz's studies and those of others that demonstrate anything to do with the validity of the energy body and energy medicine are all too often swept under the rug by mainstream science, while spectacles such as a nine-year-old girl's science fair project are willingly brought forth and applauded as "proof" that such a thing as the energy body is a figment of the imagination. The problem, then, is one of bias and the reigning paradigm. Our current paradigm of biology and medicine is still firmly entrenched in a mechanistic worldview that eschews such concepts as life energy, energy medicine, biofields, and the like, despite mounting evidence to the contrary. This is not science; this is dogmatism.

BRIDGING THE CURRENT
AND COMING PARADIGMS

How, then, do we move forward? A bridge must be built, between what is known and what is purportedly not known. Sound can potentially provide this bridge, being what we call *matter,* and *energy,* and *subtle energy.* All of these "things" are fundamentally frequency fields of energy and information, vibrating at different rates. Sound isn't either conventional or alternative—it's both. We are both a particle and a wave, a bag of biomolecules and a field of complex and varying electromagnetic frequencies.

Science currently understands how the principles of resonance and entrainment operate in music therapy, and it is a small step to see how these principles can apply to the therapeutic benefits of using tuning forks. And potentially, with some more advanced research methods, we can also clearly demonstrate this field of energy and information that surrounds the body. Once subtle energy is described, measured, and defined, we can no longer dismiss biofield therapies as having no basis in science.

The implications for this are significant. Biofield therapies are one of the most controversial and least understood therapeutic applications in complementary and alternative medicine at this time (described by some sources as a "battlefield"). The feedback loop provided by tuning forks as they pass through the biofield provides evidence of the changing terrain of this medium. Demonstrating that this field exists, appears to contain historical information in a compartmentalized fashion, and that sound intervention can effect changes in this field potentially provides a plausible explanation for how other biofield practices operate.

The acknowledgment of subtle energy—of spirit—by science is a game-changer. We can no longer call it "alternative" medicine if it is described and validated by science. We can no longer call issues that deal with subtle energy "metaphysics" or "pseudoscience." In unifying these two camps, we will have created a truly integrative, holistic worldview.

Once we have crossed this bridge, into a world of waves *and* particles instead of only particles, we have entered a domain where Biofield Tuning makes sense. And we have crossed from a cosmology of separation to one of interconnection, where we understand that treating a vibrational imbalance in any one person helps treat the imbalances in humankind—and in a very small way, the entire cosmos.

7

THE ANATOMY
OF THE BIOFIELD

Using the Chakras and
the Biofield in Sound Healing

*Informational medicine that changes disturbed
information available in the biofield is going to be
the future of medicine.*

LYNNE MCTAGGART, *THE LIVING MATRIX*

In this chapter we will go through the biofield anatomy in depth. Please refer to the Biofield Anatomy map in appendix C for a visual reference of where the issues discussed in this chapter present themselves in the biofield. I want to reiterate that this model is merely a hypothesis, one that has yet to be tested scientifically. I teach my students that when they use the biofield map, they suggest to their clients that each area *may* relate to the following areas of the body, not that it positively does relate, as I have no scientific proof of my discoveries concerning the biofields, only experiential knowledge.

We'll start at the feet and work our way up to the head. In each section we will learn the information that I have discovered in both the front and the back of the body. In this biofield model, information found at the outer edge of the field—around five feet on most people—relates to gestation, birth, and early childhood. Information found close to the body is current or recent. All other years fall in between, like rings in a tree, or light-years. As we generate the information, it moves away from us (like the way hair grows). The fields of adults and children are about the same size, but the rings get smaller as we get older. A person age forty will have information stored at the midpoint of the field (relative to the edge of the body, not the midline of the body; the biofield moves from the edge of the body outward, like tree rings); this relates to the year a forty-year-old person was about age twenty.

I have discovered that there appears to be a north-south axis as well as an east-west axis within the biofield. The north-south axis runs along the body from head to toe and appears to relate to what we understand to be the transverse waves of electromagnetism. It includes the toroidal-shaped bubble that comprises the bioplasmic body, or "soul," and is time-bound, meaning as related to the three-dimensional space-time continuum in which our human lives exist. The east-west axis runs in the direction of outstretched hands parallel to the ground. It exists within the torus but also beyond it, to infinity, and in all directions. It appears to relate to the longitudinal waves of electromagnetism, also called *Tesla waves, scalar waves, torsion waves, aether,* or even *the Higgs field.* I relate this field to "spirit," and it seems to contain, like the Akashic Records, the record of the soul's journey, perhaps through multiple lifetimes; as such it is outside of time.

I see that the bioplasmic bubble relates to plasma/bioplasma/biophotons/soul/transverse electromagnetic waves; and the underlying ground state also present relates to aether/spirit/scalar/longitudinal waves. Our human body in this lifetime appears to exist at the juncture of these two axes. It could also be called a convergence of energy and information.

The sides of each chakra are like file drawers containing records of a specific emotion or state of mind. We energize different parts of the bioplasmic body depending on what we think, feel, and experience. When we routinely spend a lot of time in a particular state of mind—for example, guilt-driven overdoing (related to the right hip)—we create an imbalance in the field that can lead to a breakdown of order, structure, and function in that region. In Biofield Tuning we are able to detect these areas of imbalance because of the perceived resistance present as reflected in the way the tone shifts in the tuning fork. We can then correct the imbalance by gently supporting the energy to return to the neutral midline down the center of the body, while modulating the tonal quality to a more balanced expression. I go into detail on the technique of using tuning forks in Biofield Tuning, as well as how to choose your tuning forks, in the next chapter. So that readers may have quick reference to a summary of each of the major chakras along with the minor knee and foot chakras, I have included two tables in appendix C (on pages 241–44).

The two tuning fork sets I previously used in Biofield Tuning are the eight-piece Solar Harmonic Spectrum set and the standard nine-piece Solfeggio set (both unweighted). The forks in the Harmonic Spectrum set are the C major scale, consisting of the octave of middle C starting at 256 Hz and ending at 512 Hz. The Solfeggio set has six original tones with both names and Hz numbers associated with them and then three additional forks that just have Hz numbers.

After years of exploration with the forks, I actually whittled down the amount of tools required, and we now make use of just three unweighted tuning forks, from the nine-piece Solfeggio set: 174 Hz, 417 Hz, and 528 Hz. However, the basic practice of field combing can really be approached with any frequency forks, though I have found just these three to be effective enough that there has been no need for more.

THE FEET

There are minor chakras present in both the feet and knees. As such, we treat them as energy centers in this method. The feet appear to contain a lot of complex information, and I have been unable to narrow them down to just a few things like I have been able to do with the rest of the body. I often come up blank when I encounter resistance around the feet; nevertheless, I have come up with a few possibilities about what information is found here.

In reflexology the feet contain the body in its entirety, so I think there is a broad range of possibilities with whatever information you may encounter around the feet. I've asked my students to pay attention to what they notice. I had one student observe that when she comes in and starts working on the feet, the distance from the body where she hits resistance will often tell her where she'll be working in the rest of the body. So if she finds resistance in the area relating to when the person was twenty years old (this distance varies depending on the age of the client), she has observed that this "tree ring" will present in other places in the body as she moves her way through. Since she mentioned this observation to me, I have also noticed the same thing.

Other things that my students have observed with regard to the feet: they are a potential link to past lives;* they relate to the energetic quality of the ground on which a person is metaphorically standing; and they represent a person's ability to support themselves (particularly the ankles) and take their next steps in life. About the latter, I have often noticed that the right foot, in particular, often contains the energy of how a person feels about their next steps. For example, if a person is nervous about what that next step might look like, there can be a sketchy or uncertain quality to the energy off the lateral (away from the midline of the body) side of this foot.

I invite you to keep an open mind while you are working around the feet and see what you notice or detect in that area. Actually, this applies to the whole body, for despite the fact that the rest of the anatomy (excluding the crown chakra) has tended to come in loud and clear to me, I would not consider my observations about the feet to be by any means definitive.

---

*Past lives are something I rarely, if ever, deal with in Biofield Tuning, simply because I prefer to deal with things that are concrete, verifiable, and able to be cross-checked, and anything that may relate to past lives can only be a matter of speculation.

THE KNEES

The left knee speaks to me of things from the past that are no longer indicated or appropriate in the present. People who resist change, who have a hard time letting go of things, whether it's a relationship or a job or things or even a story about themselves and about their lives, often hold on to "stuff" longer than is appropriate or healthy. If you find a lot of resistance in this area, the person may be spending a lot of time thinking things like, *Should I stay in this job/relationship/living situation, etc., or should I go?* Any significant stories related to this inability to release and move forward all show up in the left knee.

The right knee speaks of challenges moving forward, or obstacles within or without. These obstacles can include other people, self-sabotage, self-limiting beliefs, or simply a habit getting in the person's way. Sometimes I will find very stuck energy at the edge of the field here that can relate to a slow or complicated birth experience. It is not uncommon for people to form beliefs about their ability to move forward based on what happens at the time of birth, and perhaps surprisingly these stories tend to inform a person's entire life experience.

You will find a lot of energy laterally (to the outside) of the right knee if a person often thinks about the future and what they want to do next. For example, addicts who spend a lot of time thinking about their next fix (or drink, or cigarette) will exhibit considerable resistance here. People who are feeling stuck or uncertain tend to have a lot of energy on the sides of both knees.

If you find a lot of energy extending from the front of the knees outward, this is an indication of what I call "greener-pasture thinking." I find that in such cases the person is often projecting out into a future, one where there is more money, more freedom, a better car, a better body, a paid-off mortgage, etc. In other words, the person is not settled in the here and now; he or she is delaying happiness in the present for some imagined better future time.

Overall, the knees speak about the degree of inner and outer freedom the person is experiencing. People with energetically free knees are able to engage in what I call "spontaneous appropriate action." It's sort of like dancing, where the person moves along through life, responding in the moment to the music and the movements of the other dancers, without engaging in old stories or knee-jerk reactions—not thinking too much about the future or overplanning it. Such a person is able to release what no longer serves the purpose of living life to the fullest so as to move freely with the current of life.

ROOT CHAKRA ⁖ FIRST PLEXUS

Color: Red

Governs: Tailbone, relationship to ground, legs and feet, hip joints, pelvis

Relates to: Home life, security, tribe, right livelihood, rootedness, groundedness

Left-side imbalance: Not doing; thinking about doing but not taking action; no rubber on the road, no connection between thoughts and actions, stuckness

Right-side imbalance: Overdoing, overthinking; overactive physically, doing too much; overactive mentally, thinking too much; often guilt driven

Overall low energy: Not sleeping well, not well rested, fighting infection

Healthy/balanced: Thoughts and feelings in accord with actions; present in the now; comfortable in the home; right livelihood; high energy level

The left side of the root chakra speaks of things we want to be doing, to be, or to have, but we are not doing, being, or having them. This could be something like wanting to start one's own business and thinking about it a lot, but not taking any action—this would show up immediately off the left side of the body. An example of this from a past event could be a woman who, as a twelve-year-old girl, wanted so badly to have a horse but never got it. All that energy of desire was experienced

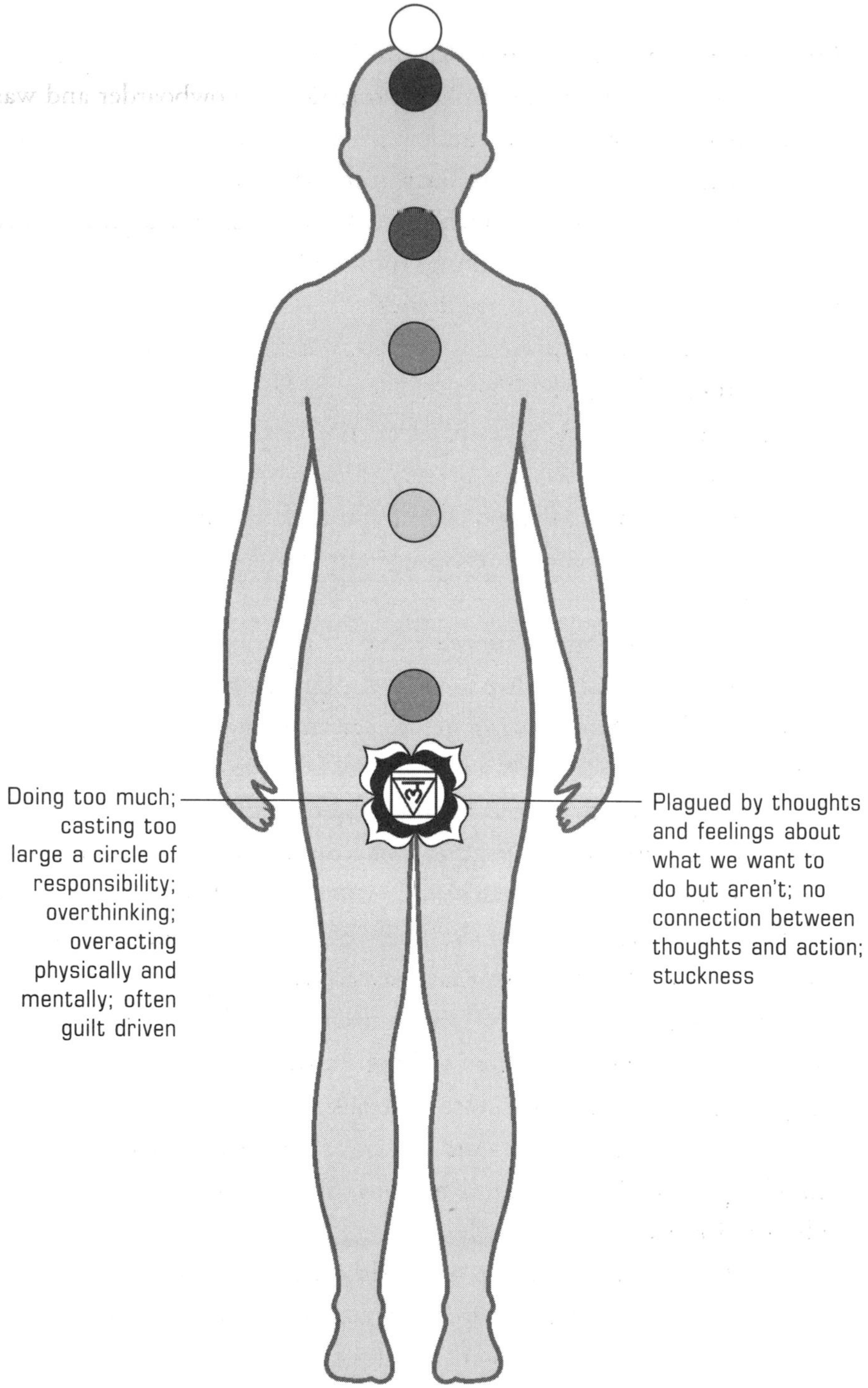

Doing too much; casting too large a circle of responsibility; overthinking; overacting physically and mentally; often guilt driven

Plagued by thoughts and feelings about what we want to do but aren't; no connection between thoughts and action; stuckness

Figure 7.1. Root Chakra—First Plexus
Home life, sense of security, groundedness

inwardly but never manifested outwardly. Another example might be a man who, as a boy, wanted to be a professional snowboarder and was good enough but lived too far away from a mountain to get there regularly, and his parents were too busy with other things to support his dream. There is a sense with energy stuck on this side that "the rubber isn't getting on the road," spinning tires, and an inability to move forward toward goals, dreams, and desires.

This is an area I often see activated in people who have eating or body-image disorders. There is a strong inclination to engage in different behavior, but an inability to do so due to the inner battle and sense of powerlessness. I recently treated two women in the same day who were both suffering from left-side sciatic pain, and they both had the same energetic imbalance in this area due to eating disorders.

I myself occasionally have left-side sciatica pain flare up, and it almost always happens when I am folding laundry—my least-favorite chore. I would rather be doing just about anything other than folding laundry.

The right side of the root chakra speaks of being busy, but not necessarily doing the things we want to be doing. A person who is very busy will have a lot of resistance around this hip. There is another key place, about fourteen to eighteen inches off the side of the body on the right side, which I call "busy mind" (see figure 7.2 on page 138). This is something found in almost everyone except for skilled meditators. And even meditators can have what I call the "meditators' paradox," whereby the person knows how to go into spaciousness and presence, but when not meditating that person's mind is just as busy as anyone else's. In the biofield, part of the busy-mind region is spacious and another part is full of resistance.

The busy mind shows up as a fairly profound imbalance in the energy body. Pioneering health-care practitioner and biophoton investigator Johan Boswinkel calls thinking "a psychological disease." The reality is that most thinking is nonproductive, nonbeneficial looping that involves worrying about the future, to-do lists, concern about

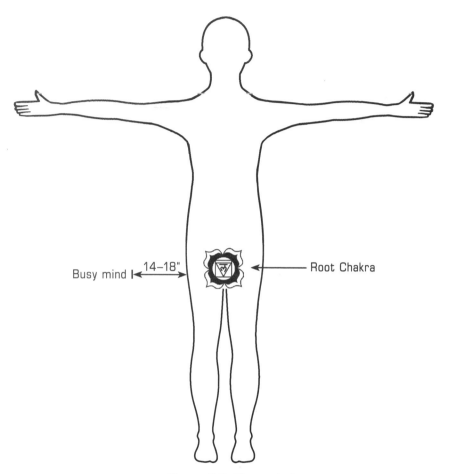

Figure 7.2. Busy mind

what other people think, inner judgment, guilt, and self-criticism. Most modern Westerners mentally beat themselves up on a regular basis, and while they might extend compassion to the people around them, they seem unable to include themselves in that equation. Most people also find it impossible to quiet their minds. The mind just goes and goes, like a wild horse. This prevents people from being in the present and wastes a lot of energy. This, to me, is one of the biggest problems of our times—that people don't know how to turn their minds off.

Just inside the busy-mind region is the busy-body region, which occupies the distance from the surface of the body to about twelve or so inches out. This is an area that will be energized if the person is always in motion. People who have a lot of energy in this area are often trying to avoid their feelings, often feelings of sadness. As long as they stay in motion, they stay out in front of their feelings, which tend to settle on them when they stop, so they keep going. I recently ran into a friend whom I hadn't seen in a while who was limping and using a cane. I asked him what was going on, and he said that he had to get his right hip replaced. I said to him, "Ah, the hip of chronic overdoing," and he said, "Exactly—I've been overdoing my whole life." So here he was, only sixty years old and he had worn out his right hip. People who are very busy will often end up with right-hip issues, including sciatica and arthritis.

The back of the root chakra speaks to me of our physical home. If there is a lot of static or a diminished tone here, it usually relates to some kind of stress regarding the home: a renovation, clutter, needing but not being able to afford a new roof (or floor or drywall repair— that sort of thing), an uncomfortable roommate situation, having to move, etc.

The back of the root chakra can also speak of a tailbone injury, which will show up as static even many years after the injury occurred. I recently worked with a woman who suffered a tailbone accident while snowboarding. She had just moved to a new home, had two small children, and had to do the lion's share of the domestic work because her husband was busy working. She was exhausted from doing way too much but was determined to get out and have some fun. The accident pushed her tailbone over toward the right, where the bulk of her root energy had shifted to (i.e., the overdoing side) while jamming it up into the sacrum, resulting in swelling and pain in her left sacral area (i.e., frustration). There is no doubt that she was very frustrated from overdoing around the home, and the pattern of her accident revealed exactly this.

SACRAL CHAKRA ⭲⭰ SECOND PLEXUS

Color: Orange

Governs: Reproductive organs, bladder, large intestine, small
intestine

Relates to: Sexuality, creativity, cash flow, self-worth,
intimate relationships

Left-side imbalance: Frustration, disappointment

Right-side imbalance: Guilt, shame

Overall low energy: Creatively stuck, unhealthy intimate
relationships, low self-worth

Healthy/balanced: Healthy intimate relationships, creatively
flowing

The left side of the sacral chakra speaks to me of frustration, and sometimes disappointment shows up here as well. It's often coupled with the
root chakra, so we end up frustrated over not doing what we want to be
doing. Frustration arises in the gap between our expectations of people,
events, or life situations, and how they really are. When we resist what
is, we are frustrated. We then put energy (in the form of the emotion
of frustration) into what we don't want instead of what we do want.
Sometimes we can feel frustrated about a situation but keep pushing
that feeling down instead of recognizing it and allowing it to move us
into a more contented and balanced place.

I recently worked with someone who is a classic "nice guy."
Whenever he felt frustrated he would push the feeling down and just
keep on being a nice guy. He had this great big bubble of energy that
was all shunted to the left side of his second chakra. All that life force,
all that vital energy, was not being engaged in his life experience. The
second chakra speaks of creativity, sexuality, and self-worth; it's a res-
ervoir of personal power, and to have it caught up in frustration, or as
we see on the other side, guilt and shame, is to be not accessing all of
one's personal power. In his case, when the energy was brought into
balance, it was very strong. He suddenly understood why other people

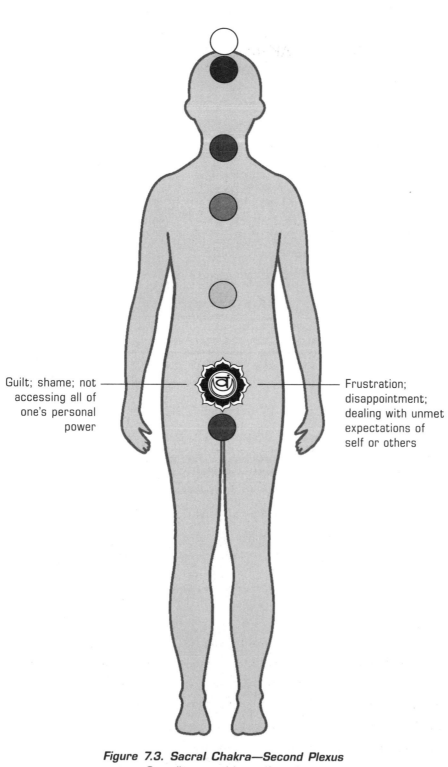

Guilt; shame; not accessing all of one's personal power

Frustration; disappointment; dealing with unmet expectations of self or others

Figure 7.3. Sacral Chakra—Second Plexus
Sexuality, creativity, self-worth

were always trying to put him into positions of leadership that he didn't feel worthy of, deferring to others instead. After this pattern shifted he began to feel much more comfortable in leadership roles and experienced a lot less frustration.

Any emotion we repress will suck a lot of juice out of us, depleting energy from the body's systems. There is the energy of the emotion itself, and then there is the energy required to keep it repressed. I often come across constructs I call "walls," which appear to be high-energy frequency barriers that block the perception of the conscious mind from "going there." When we use sound to deconstruct those constructs, to free up that energy and then give it back to the system as a whole, we suddenly have reserves of energy that we didn't have before to get things done.

Since the energetic field is the "exploded" view of the body, and the life situation/home is the exploded view of that, these pockets of congestion in a person's field often correspond to pockets of physical clutter or chaos in that person's environment—as within, so without. Once a person has order in that part of the signaling that had previously been characterized by disorder and noise, the associated outer reflection of clutter or chaos in the person's environment usually disappears. It is not unusual in such a case that the person goes home from a session and cleans out all her closets, tackling piles of stuff she hadn't had the energy to tackle previously.

One interesting thing I have found on the left side of the second chakra is resistance at the outer edge of the field if the person was bottle-fed instead of breastfed. These persons often suffered frequent stomachaches as young children and may even have had digestive issues right up to the present. Some people who are allergic or sensitive to dairy products rarely if ever connect it to the fact that they were bottle-fed as infants. I have worked with many people who have gone through powerful detox experiences as a result of working with sound on this issue, and they subsequently enjoyed much better and more efficient digestion as a result.

The right side of the second chakra speaks of guilt or shame. Guilt and shame are similar but different. The simplest distinction between the two that I have ever heard is that guilt is reflected in the statement "I did something bad," whereas shame is "I am bad." Psychiatrist and spiritual teacher David Hawkins, in his book *Power vs Force*, says that of all the possible human emotions, shame is the heaviest, the lowest on the frequency scale. Shame is a very difficult emotion to feel because it feels so terrible, and so what a lot of people do instead of feeling that feeling is repress it and then displace it onto others through finger-pointing and blame.

Blaming other people instead of feeling shame is a very common phenomenon, particularly among alcoholics, and there tends to be a lot of repressed emotions in this area. In fact, this area is jam-packed with so much stuck "stuff" in just about everyone that it's almost ridiculous.

One of the things that I have encountered in this area is what I call the *slavery yoke,* which is another term for what Sol Luckman, a visual artist and author of fiction and nonfiction, has identified as the *fragmentary body* in his book *Potentiate Your DNA*. There appears to be some kind of energetic construct built into our fields that keeps our vital life energy eddying in these bottom two chakras instead of rising up into and through the crown. I know this sounds kind of far-out, but bear with me, because it potentially explains a lot.

As I said previously, the root and second chakras are coupled, and a pattern you find in one is almost always connected to a pattern in the other. Because of the insertion of something like an energetic barrier that appears to lie in the region between the second and third chakras, like a disc parallel to the ground, life energy gets trapped in the two bottom chakras. The result is either guilt- and shame-driven overdoing, or frustrated nondoing, or a pattern of going back and forth between the two. Either way, people accumulate heavy imbalances in this part of their fields (see figure 7.4 on page 144).

In the months leading up to taking the time to write this book, I found myself becoming increasingly intolerant of the busy, guilty-mind energy spinning in people's fields, about eighteen inches off

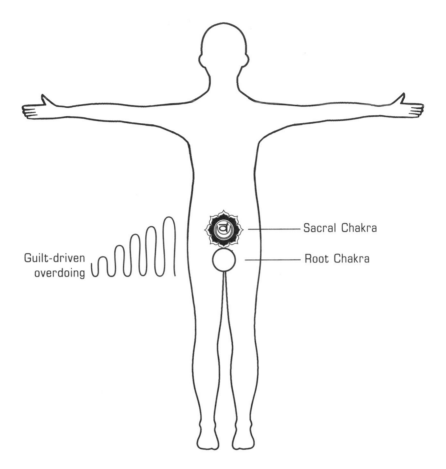

Figure 7.4. Guilt-driven overdoing

the right hip. People's minds spin and spin with voices they cannot silence—a punishing inner critic, a never-ending to-do list, an inability to rest or feel worthy unless they are being productive. While I usually am quite patient and neutral in sessions, there was something about finding this spiraling, stuck energy in everyone that started to bother me more and more.

At first I didn't understand why. As the saying goes, we tend to dislike in others what we dislike in ourselves, but initially I did not see the connection. A big part of this spin is the "inner critic" who beats up on herself with admonishments of imperfection and inadequacy. In my conscious mind, this was not something that I did; in fact, I had been under the impression that I had silenced the inner critic and had learned to tame my busy mind years ago. It was easy for me to quiet my thoughts, to go into spaciousness and inner silence, I thought. So why was this bothering me so much?

The answer came from a couple of different sources. One, it dawned on me that what was not quiet in me was my inner to-do list. I was superwoman: wife, mom, teacher, therapist, school-board member, researcher, book writer. I was a perpetual motion machine, a veritable pinball of kinetic energy, but I had it in my head that since I had mastered the twenty-minute power nap, I was good at "just being." I didn't see the frenetic quality in my own mind because I was so accustomed to it. Because I couldn't see it in myself, I was starting to feel frustrated when I saw it in others, and I was becoming increasingly intolerant of it.

Another source of information that answered my question came from a healing process I had experienced a few months earlier called Potentiation, a technique pioneered by the previously mentioned Sol Luckman. Potentiation is a therapeutic treatment brilliantly uncovered by Sol and his partner, Leigh, that uses the MI Solfeggio fork with a frequency of 528 Hz and specifically intoned vowels to recode one's DNA to change its expression. Sol describes it as the ninth chakra descending and sealing the fragmentary body, or what I call the "slavery yoke." This then allows energy to start flowing up into the rest of the energy body more readily. Sol says that before this sealing takes place, the body is pushing out all kinds of toxins, including parasites that can accumulate in our bodies because of this barrier to proper circulation.

In the process of this energy shift taking place in me I suddenly started to see things that I had previously been blind to. One of the exercises that proved very helpful with this was the question, "What are properties of mine that I regularly feel an aversion to?" Remember, I was under the conscious impression that I had silenced the inner critic and was pretty much having love and compassion for myself. Not so! I filled a half a page quickly in answer to this question—I was subconsciously beating myself up all over the place. Guilt is something that often runs subconsciously—we feel guilty and inadequate regularly, but it is so common and "normal" that we don't even perceive it. And even though I was very aware of this fact, I was still doing it myself. It took asking the right question for the pattern to finally be revealed. Once I became aware of it, I was able to notice it as it arose—not to stop the judgment, because that is not so easy to do at first, but to extend compassion through the judgment.

Not to stereotype, but I often find that people raised in homes that were orthodox Catholic or Jewish seem to have large amounts of guilt in their fields. Other sorts of things that show up in this area relate to sexuality—sexual abuse, abortions, even difficult pregnancies and births imprint their record in this region. Having large amounts of energy stuck in the field on either side of the second chakra can be very disempowering and even paralyzing, especially when it comes to creativity.

I highly recommend Sol's books *Potentiate Your DNA* and *Conscious Healing.* In *Potentiate Your DNA,* he gives instructions on how you can seal your own fragmentary body, as well as those of others, if you choose to. If you don't want to take the time to learn the method, you can receive the process from Sol or one of the facilitators he has trained at the Phoenix Center of Regenetics. I think this work is very complementary to the Biofield Tuning process. In Sol's words, "Sound healing is the frontier of true holistic medicine, for sound gives us access to the quantum realm of bioenergy and empowers us to consciously modify our quantum biology for personal (and even planetary) healing and transformation."[1]

SOLAR PLEXUS CHAKRA ⇥⇤ THIRD PLEXUS

Color: Yellow

Governs: Spleen, pancreas, stomach, kidneys, adrenals, liver, gallbladder; also relationship with mother and father

Relates to: Self-confidence, self-esteem, how we interface
with others' energies, setting goals and achieving them
Left-side imbalance: Powerlessness
Right-side imbalance: Anger
Overall low energy: Not assertive, challenged by setting and
achieving goals, easily overwhelmed by others' energy
Healthy/balanced: Assertive, able to advocate for self, able
to complete projects

The third chakra is an incredibly complex area, containing so much information that it seems to me that there may even be another electromagnetic axis of sorts here. It contains information related to mother, father, anger, powerlessness, and the kidneys, adrenals, spleen, pancreas, liver, gallbladder, and stomach. Being able to determine exactly what you are encountering as you work in this area requires deep listening and a lot of hands-on hours. I have learned how to differentiate between all of these aspects, but this ability has evolved over time. I describe it to my students as being like learning a new language. You gradually learn new words, and once you know a new word, it becomes part of your vocabulary, and you recognize it and understand it when you hear it. It is like that with learning to distinguish what vibrational information is coming from the body the loudest and strongest in that particular moment. You will have "ah-ha" moments, just as I have, when you suddenly learn the difference between the physical level and the emotional level, or what scar tissue sounds like, or what fear sounds like.

This is an area that students have pushed me to describe with more detail, but the process is so subtle that it is often beyond words. I can only tell you to become quiet inside, listen closely, and trust what you hear and feel. That is all I have ever done, and hopefully I have made it clear thus far that I have no special gifts beyond what anyone else has in this department; in fact, I have had to work hard to be able to hear clearly in my life.

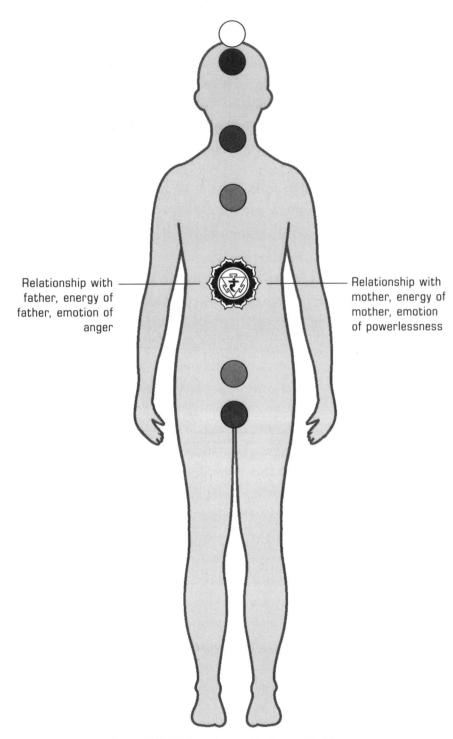

Relationship with father, energy of father, emotion of anger

Relationship with mother, energy of mother, emotion of powerlessness

Figure 7.5. Solar Plexus Chakra—Third Plexus
Self-confidence, interacting with others' energy, setting and achieving goals

The Left Side:
Spleen, Pancreas, Stomach, Kidneys, Adrenals, Mother

The left side of the solar plexus speaks to me of a person's relationship with the mother from conception until the present. This can also be stepmother, adoptive mother, or grandmother if this applies. This place also holds the energy of the mother herself, about ten to twelve inches off the left side of the body. When I have the fork vibrating in this specific area, I can generally tell with accuracy the temperament or personality of the mother, as this energy shows up very distinctly.

If people had difficult relationships with their mothers when they were infants or babies, if there was a lot of chaos or a failure to bond, there will be a lot of resistance in the outer edge of the field in this region. Often one finds resistance in the area of adolescence (the location for this differs depending on age), especially in women—the age of fourteen to sixteen seems to be a common time for girls and their mothers to have a lot of stress between them.

If there is a lot of energy over the body itself toward the left side of the chakra—for example, over the area of the spleen or pancreas—I have found that this relates to an inability to nourish oneself properly or to make choices that are supportive of one's well-being. This can relate to physical health: say, if a person is a smoker and wants to quit but keeps choosing cigarettes anyway, or if he is eating poorly and would perhaps prefer to make better choices, that misdirected energy seems to accumulate here. In trying to boil down the phenomenon to just one word, I come up with *powerlessness.*

When we are unable to make the best choices for ourselves in the moment, whether that means standing up for ourselves in a social situation or picking nourishing food or going to bed at a reasonable hour, whether we do this by habit or by a tendency to go unconscious, all of this points to an inability to feel empowered in that moment to choose what best serves us. This tendency is often tied in to how we were nourished or not nourished by our mothers.

The adrenals are small glands roughly the size of a walnut, which sit on top of each kidney. They produce the hormones adrenaline (also known as *epinephrine*) and cortisol. Adrenaline is produced under periods of high stress when we need a burst of energy, whereas cortisol is produced throughout the day and also helps the body regulate the stress of everyday living. Cortisol in too great an amount, as a consequence of long-term, low-level stress, becomes detrimental if it accumulates in the body.

Adrenal fatigue from both intense periodic and chronic low-level stressors is an enormous issue in our culture. One of the very exciting things about Biofield Tuning is the ability of sound to influence what I call the "adrenal rhythm." This is exactly what it sounds like—a happy adrenal produces a good, normal, healthy rhythm, but a stressed adrenal makes a lot of noise. This noise affects the whole body, like the way a car alarm going off outside your window might affect you. Nothing functions well under stress.

I have been surprised to discover that each adrenal appears to react to different stressors, and as such I have given them each a name. The left adrenal appears to be stimulated when we are in acute pain or under a physical stressor, where we might need to fight or flee—I call it the "saber-toothed tiger" adrenal. The right adrenal appears to be stimulated when we are under social stress, whether at home or at work; there's no threat to our physical well-being, but we are acutely stressed regardless. I call this one the "office-politics" adrenal.

Generally, I encounter a lot more right adrenal issues than left. But if someone is in an abusive relationship, an unsafe neighborhood, or a dangerous vocation, the left adrenal also will run like a toilet with a stuck handle. I recently worked with a woman in her mid-sixties and was surprised to find a "thumping" left adrenal, and when I told her that this one usually behaved that way when under physical threat, she informed me that she had had a run-in with a group of teenagers in her neighborhood, including one who had gotten in her face in her own driveway. She lived on a cul-de-sac and no longer felt safe in her own neighborhood. This woman had also just gotten out of a job that had been very stressful, with considerable tension between herself and her boss, and her right adrenal was also on high alert.

The abusive or dangerous relationship can also be with oneself. Many people continue a parent's or sibling's habit of attacking, even after they no longer come in contact with the perpetrator, by attacking oneself.

When adrenaline is constantly being released into the system, it seems to me as if the other energy-production systems of the body take a backseat. When I reset a person's adrenal glands, bringing them back to neutral, the person will generally have a one- to three-day period where he feels completely exhausted. This seems to be a recalibration of sorts as the rest of the body comes back online. Once the energy returns, the person feels much better than before. It is very important to rest during this time of recalibration, to stay well hydrated, and trust that energy will return.

Right Side: Liver, Gallbladder, Kidneys, Adrenals, Father, Anger

The right side of the third chakra relates to father and one's relationship with father and also to the emotion of anger. The liver stores and metabolizes anger. Many people who had or still have difficult relationships with their fathers (stepfathers, adopted fathers, grandfathers) have a tendency to repress the difficult feelings associated with this by engaging in consumption of what I call "liver pacifiers": sugar, excessive amounts of carbs, alcohol, chocolate, and dense dairy products such as ice cream or cheese. Obviously, in small amounts these substances are fine, but in excess they have the effect of dampening or even eliminating our experience of anger (the "angry drunk" would be an exception to this).

One of the things that I have been consistently surprised to come across is just how many issues people seem to have with their fathers. Having been raised in a culture that taught me about Freud and the notion that everything is the fault of the mother (I know that this is a simplification of Freud, but it is definitely the perception that I and many others ended up with), I did not expect to find a greater amount of father issues in people than mother issues. It seems that many dads are/were alcoholics, rageaholics, workaholics, emotionally unavailable, in prison, or just not around or otherwise present to their child's needs. The fundamental things that people seem to need from their fathers—acknowledgment, approval, and affection—are rarely if ever received, and this seems to give rise to some real problems for people. (Remember the demographic here: people seeking help in dealing with issues, not necessarily the population at large.)

In the absence of the reflection of our own inner brilliance that a healthy relationship with one's father can provide, many people end up unconsciously seeking to get these needs met as they go through their lives, engaging in guilt-driven overdoing, experiencing feelings of low self-worth, seeking approval, and routinely putting others' needs ahead of their own.

In addition to the relationship with and the character of the father, the right side of the third chakra also holds the energy of the liver. In my years of working with sound, I have come to have a great appreciation of the liver. In Chinese medicine the liver is seen as the general in the army that is the body; it is responsible for overseeing all operations. The liver pays attention to digestion, respiration, circulation, subtle-energy flow, elimination, the immune function, and probably more things besides. People debate as to whether the seat of consciousness is in the heart or the brain, but I have started to see it as being in the liver.

Also, in Chinese medicine it is said that the liver opens to the eyes, and we say that the eyes are the windows to the soul. If you or anyone you know has ever done a liver cleanse, you know how clear and bright the eyes become afterward. The liver is also the organ of discernment—it decides what in the self needs to be recycled and what is to be disposed of. This quality of discernment is such a big part of what makes us individuals. And in traditional hunting societies, the liver of wild game is highly prized for its abundance of life force.

I did an internet search of "the seat of consciousness is in the liver" and found that the discovery of the importance of the brain as the seat of thought and action was not part of human knowledge until barely two centuries ago. Apparently, the heart, the navel, and the liver have all been revered by different cultures at different times as the seat of consciousness.[2] The ancient Greeks in particular ascribed consciousness as arising from the liver. Regardless of what the truth may be—likely a triad of the heart, brain, and liver—the liver is an incredibly important organ, one that is, unfortunately, under massive assault in modern times. There have been an enormous amount of toxins put into circulation in the last hundred years or so—so many toxic chemicals have been released into the air, the earth, and the water that our bodies are under continual assault. Our homes, our clothes, our cars, our offices are all teeming with chemicals that the human liver never had to deal with even just a few generations ago. Widespread alcohol and drug use, both pharmaceutical and street, along with genetically modified foods, pesticides and herbicides, artificial colorings and flavorings, BPA and other plastics—the list goes on and on—all lead to a very difficult time for our livers, and consequently for our consciousness. Add the pollution of television, radio, electromagnetic radiations of all sorts, and the dissonance of a lot of popular music, and it's a wonder any of us are healthy at all.

Another key pollutant and obscurant to liver health is the emotion of anger. I'll talk more about the concept of "purplewashing," or suppressing our emotions, in chapter 9, but briefly, the emotion of anger—the electrochemical peptide that holds the information of that emotion—appears to be stored in the liver. When people suppress or deny or stuff their anger, it accumulates here, where it inhibits optimum functioning.

I once worked with a woman whose now ex-husband was an alcoholic who had continually made bad choices that had a negative impact on her. Wanting to be nice, compassionate, and understanding, she had buried huge amounts of anger under a several-glasses-of-wine-a-night habit. The image that came to mind when I was working on her liver was of a dumpster that had not been emptied in a long time and was piled up with garbage on top of and all around it. Biofield Tuning can stimulate significant detox, and this was one of those times. Because the woman was otherwise very healthy, I worked deeply with the energy of her liver and informed her that she would most likely experience some uncomfortable detox symptoms. Over the next few days she had bouts of fever and developed a skin rash—a classic healing crisis wherein her body was eliminating the toxins that had been held in the liver field and were now exiting. After this she found it easier to get in touch with and deal with her anger instead of masking it.

I haven't learned a lot about the gallbladder, which connects to the liver, pancreas, and duodenum of the small intestine, although I have speculated that it too may relate to upset or anger over lack of support by the father. I have observed this common denominator in clients I have had who have had their gallbladders removed.

In Chinese medicine the kidneys are said to store shock and fear. I have found this on occasion, but not as a rule. Fear, like anxiety, seems to be free-floating to me, meaning I can find it in just about any chakra, depending on what it is related to. Different people experience fear-based anxiety in different parts of their bodies—it could be the knees, the lower abdomen, the solar plexus, chest, throat, or in the head. The emotion may be radiating or referring from the kidney region, although this is not something I have observed.

Anxiety is an interesting frequency in the body. To me, it seems like it is more of a feeling than an emotion—specifically, the feeling of an emotion trying to rise up and push itself into our awareness and the feeling of our awareness trying to suppress the feeling, thus creating an uncomfortable agitation. I often ask people who suffer from chronic anxiety, "What is the emotion that is under your anxiety?" and they will often be surprised to discover that once they allow themselves to really feel whatever feeling that is, the anxiety diminishes. Sometimes it isn't even something that may be perceived as negative—I have had many people report that they discovered emotions like excitement under their anxiety.

The Mother and Father Zones

There is a fixed space in the region of the third chakra, about ten inches away from the body on each side, which holds the energy of the mother on the left and the father on the right (see figure 7.6). These energies cannot be moved, but any discord in these spots can be balanced and integrated. I am able to tell a lot about the personality and energies of the parent by what I find here and also about the dynamics between the person and the parent.

One of the things that has amazed me is how people's relationships with their parents can really change and shift through Biofield Tuning. I have heard over and over again from clients upon returning from visits with parents after a Biofield Tuning treatment that their buttons weren't pushed, that they were able to be peaceable and proactive with parents who had previously been very difficult to be around. I have even

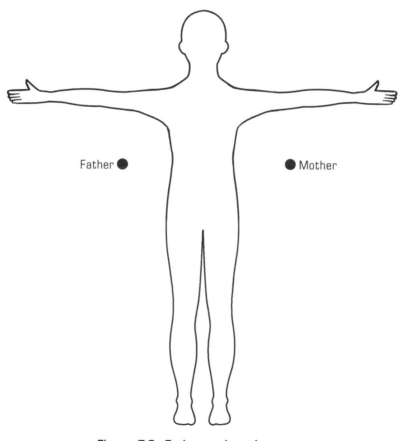

Father ●   ● Mother

Figure 7.6. Father and mother zones,
fixed spots approximately ten inches from the body

had clients report seeing significant changes in their parents after being around them—the work seems to "go upstream" and affect the energy of the parent in subtle but often tangible ways.

The back of the solar plexus relates to issues of support: the degree to which we were supported or unsupported by our parents, the degree to which we are able to support ourselves, both physically and emotionally, and the degree of support we receive, or allow ourselves to receive, from others. If there is pain in this area, it is often the case that the person is supporting others but doesn't have anyone who's got their back.

HEART CHAKRA ›‹ FOURTH PLEXUS

Color: Green
Governs: Heart, lungs
Relates to: Giving and receiving love, compassion, and gratitude
Left-side imbalance: Sadness, grief, and loss
Right-side imbalance: Saying yes when we mean no, overdoing for others
Overall low energy: Challenge to give and receive love, harboring old pain, suffering from depression
Healthy/balanced: Following heart's desires, able to love freely

The first area I ever identified in the biofield anatomy was the left side of the heart chakra, when I realized that I kept finding sad stories in this area. Sadness is a very easy emotion to recognize through tuning fork overtones because it sounds very much like the way sad music sounds. There is no mistaking sadness. Energy blips show up here as a result of the deaths of loved ones or pets; moving, especially as children; being ignored, abused, or neglected; the ending of a relationship; and even the death of dreams.

If a person suffers from depression or is frequently sad, you will find a lot of energy just off the left shoulder. Left-shoulder issues often arise

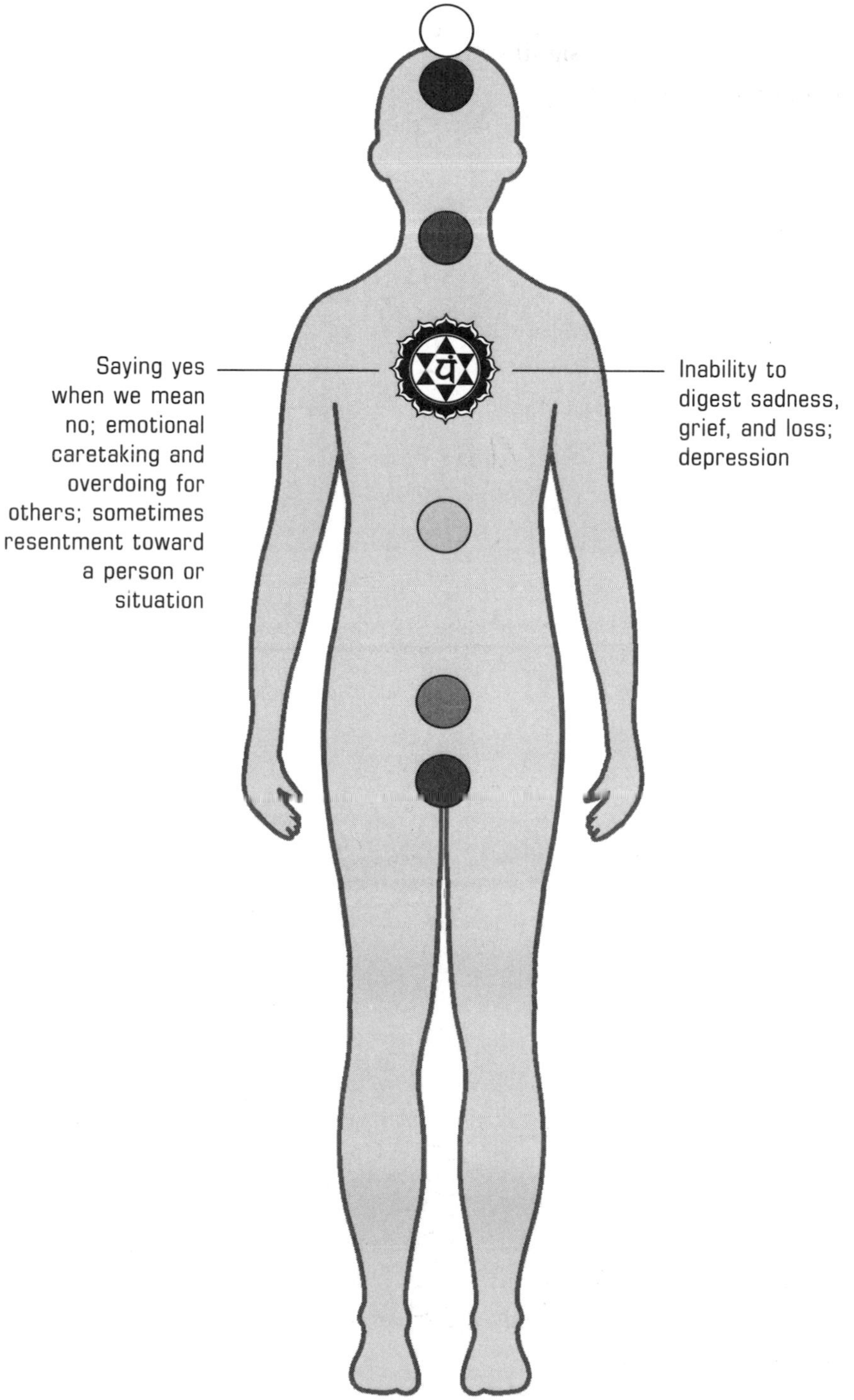

Saying yes when we mean no; emotional caretaking and overdoing for others; sometimes resentment toward a person or situation

Inability to digest sadness, grief, and loss; depression

Figure 7.7. Heart Chakra—Fourth Plexus
Giving and receiving love, compassion, and gratitude

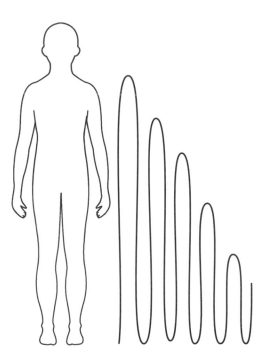

Figure 7.8. Left-hand ditch—frustrated, sad, and stuck energy, often a consequence of lack of support from the mother

from undigested or unprocessed sadness that is weighing on the person. I often see a constellation of stuck energy that I call the "left-hand ditch," where there is a lot of sadness and frustration present, often from a lack of early support from the mother (see figure 7.8).

The right side of the heart chakra relates to saying yes when we mean no, or putting other people's needs or expectations ahead of our own natural inclinations (see figure 7.9). While helping others can be a source of great joy, when we do it continuously, especially when we do it while going against a strong inner "no," we do ourselves a great disservice. Many people get into this habit because they want to be loved or accepted. It is also a habit I see strongly in oldest children, especially in larger families, because in many cases they were routinely expected to help with younger siblings. I also see it in people who were unsupported in childhood in their dreams and desires, who developed a kind of "I'm not worthy of what I want so I might as well just help others get what they want" attitude.

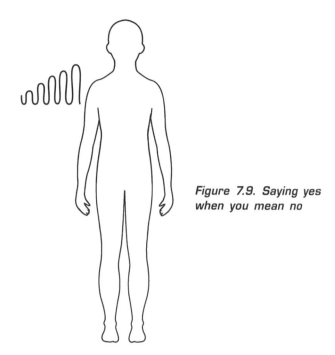

Figure 7.9. Saying yes when you mean no

I sometimes call this the "nice girl" or "yes man" shoulder, as these are the people who often end up with issues here. Many people who end up in the healing arts have this helper personality profile, and I have worked on many a massage therapist with right-shoulder issues. Another reason this attitude is so widespread comes from the cultural edict of "service above self," where we are taught that doing what we want to do, looking after our own needs and wants, is selfish and unacceptable. While it is indeed noble to serve humanity, doing it to the detriment of our own health and well-being serves no one in the end, because a routine habit of this breaks down our health to the point where we may end up needing caretaking ourselves.

Every client I have ever worked with who had fibromyalgia has had large amounts of stuck energy in this area. The fibromyalgia personality has usually spent a lifetime putting everyone else's needs ahead of their own until their body reaches a point where it rebels and starts refusing to do anything. They become so stuffed with resentment and frustration and undigested emotion that their circuits become over-loaded. I have found it is helpful for these people to start speaking and standing up for themselves when it is appropriate to do so.

The back of the heart speaks of love we receive from others and the degree to which we let it in or hold it back. Trigger points around the left shoulder blade can speak of defending ourselves against someone else's negative energy, and this develops when we clench this area to protect the back of the physical and energetic heart. Trigger points around the right shoulder blade can speak of holding back aggressive or angry thoughts or feelings.

Lower trigger points that fall midway between the heart and the solar plexus chakras can speak of sadness and/or anger over a lack of support, from the father on the right or the mother on the left.

THROAT CHAKRA ⋙⋘ FIFTH PLEXUS

Color: Blue
Governs: Thyroid, jaw, throat, faculty of hearing
Relates to: Communication, speaking one's truth, creativity
Left-side imbalance: Not communicating or expressing, holding back
Right-side imbalance: Speaking and not being heard
Overall low energy: Not expressing self, thyroid issues, holding back
Healthy/balanced: Communicating clearly, being heard, particularly strong energy relates to teacher, writer, or other communication vocation

The left side of the throat chakra speaks of that which we do not say or express. People who are in the habit of not speaking their truth, not sharing their feelings or perspective, or not standing up for themselves will accumulate energy on the left side of the throat. The throat chakra is often coupled with the heart chakra, just like the first and second chakras are often coupled, so if a person has not allowed

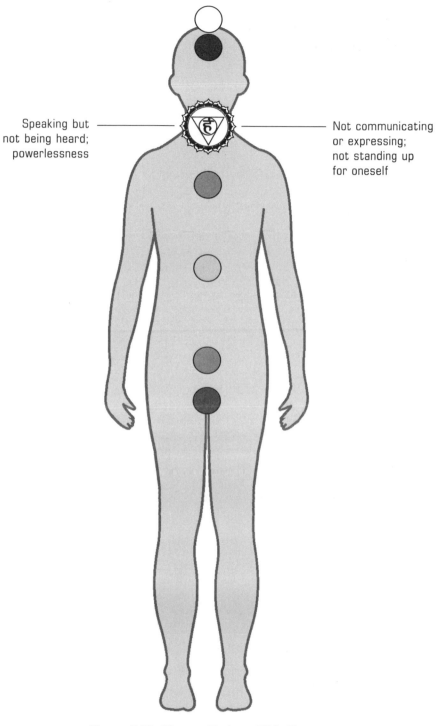

Speaking but not being heard; powerlessness

Not communicating or expressing; not standing up for oneself

Figure 7.10. Throat Chakra—Fifth Plexus
Communication, speaking our truth, creativity

herself to feel or express her sadness, you will usually find pockets of dual-chakra unexpressed and undigested sadness. The impulse to express something is an electromagnetic event, and if it is suppressed, it accumulates, it builds up, and energy that is built up like this creates inflammation. It is very important to express these energies. "Better out than in!" is one of the profound truths I have seen in this work.

The right side of the throat chakra speaks to me of speaking but not being heard. People with stuck energy here, especially about six to eight inches off the right side of the body, are often engaged in a relationship where there is a lot of arguing going on. We all know that when we are in a heated argument, nobody gets anywhere because we are refusing to see the value and validity of the perspective of the person we are arguing with, just as the other person is refusing to validate us. (Remember the metaphor of truth having 144 sides in the introduction to this book.) We may have this kind of relationship with our kids, our boss, our neighbors, our siblings, or our parents, where it doesn't matter what we say, nobody is listening or responding or validating us. This is the ultimate in powerlessness. It is by being heard and responded to that we are powerful, that we influence the world around us. Powerful people are people who are heard and respected by many other people. Powerless people have no voice.

I have said many times that the throat chakra is the most important chakra that I work on. It is by our words that we create our lives, and if we do not express the words that our hearts and minds generate, then we are not creating authentic lives. People tend to get caught up in dualistic thinking when it comes to self-expression, thinking *I am either a good girl or a bitch,* or *I'm either a nice guy or a jerk,* when in fact there is a functional, peaceable, diplomatic middle path. It can take a little while to master this middle road, especially if a person has spent a lifetime either saying nothing at all or telling other people what they want to hear. Truthful diplomacy is a learned skill, but almost without exception I have seen people who have undergone Biofield Tuning learn to advocate for themselves successfully and start to create more authentic, real, and ultimately less stressful life situations for themselves.

Thyroid function is also governed by the energy of the throat chakra. Very often people with under- or overactive thyroids have energetic imbalances in their throat chakras, and I have seen several instances where people either reduced or got off their thyroid medication altogether after receiving Biofield Tuning.

Neck stiffness or soreness can be related to the above energetic issues, but I have also observed many cases where a person's neck goes out of alignment to the point where she needs regular chiropractic adjustment, especially during times of stress, when I have traced the origin of it back to a physical accident the person had when they were quite young—as young as four or even younger. Sledding accidents, head injuries, car accidents, and other whiplash-inducing experiences can create torque in the field that will keep pulling the body out of alignment. Often, after the energy is released through Biofield Tuning, the body will stop going out as much, many times resolving completely.

The back of the throat chakra seems to relate to our ability to channel inspiration. I have seen many instances where once this area is opened up energetically, the person has an easier time writing or singing songs, has greater spontaneity and freedom of expression in writing and speaking, or senses a greater connection to their own intuitive guidance.

THIRD EYE CHAKRA ⇒⇐ SIXTH PLEXUS

Color: Purple or indigo
Governs: Pineal gland, brain
Relates to: Intuition, thought processes
Left-side imbalance: Worrying about the future
Right-side imbalance: Overthinking about the past
Overall low energy: Inability to focus, distrust or
   disconnection from intuition

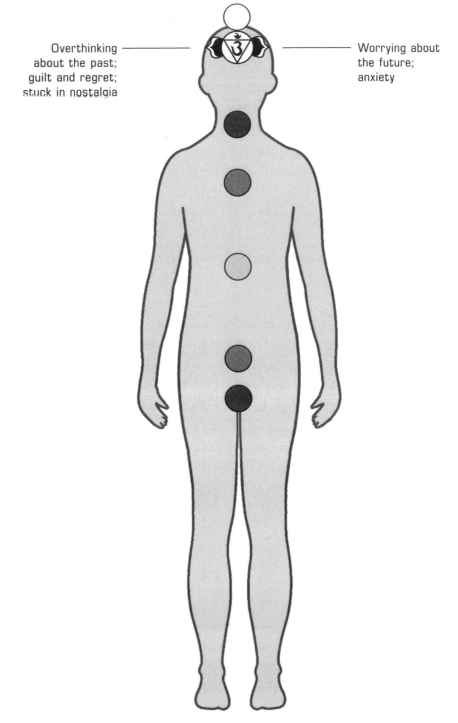

Overthinking about the past; guilt and regret; stuck in nostalgia

Worrying about the future; anxiety

Figure 7.11. Third Eye Chakra—Sixth Plexus
Intuition, thought processes

Healthy/balanced: Clear third eye perception, mental focus and acuity

The left side of the sixth chakra speaks to me of worry about the future. There is an area approximately eight inches off the side of the head that I call "the hamster wheel of worry." This is the place that gets energized when you start thinking about the future and wondering how you are going to pay your bills, provide for your children's college education, what you are going to say to so-and-so, how you are going to manage dealing with a boss or coworker, and so on. Thoughts that run here are often anxiety- and tension-producing: anxious anticipation of potential future events.

The right side of the sixth chakra speaks to me of thoughts about the past. These are often fraught with guilt and regret but can also be reflections on the positive or "good old days." If there is an event from a person's life to which he goes back over and over again in his thinking, this particular area in the timeline will be charged.

PTSD Head

This is the best name I have been able to come up with so far to describe the phenomenon of charge around the head of a person who has PTSD, or post-traumatic stress disorder, an anxiety disorder that may develop after a person is exposed to one or more traumatic events, such as sexual assault, serious injury, warfare, or the threat of death. With this you will encounter thick energy and static from the edge of the field all the way to the head, usually on both sides (see figure 7.12 on page 166). I describe it as being like a large house with every light and appliance turned on in every room. There is so much neural activity that the person can barely handle any more input because there is no available brain area or energy to process it.

PTSD is one of the areas where I have seen near-miraculous outcomes as a result of Biofield Tuning. The sound acts as if it turns off the lights and appliances and turns down the noise in the brain, allowing for normal processing of stimuli and the ability to resume more normal functioning.

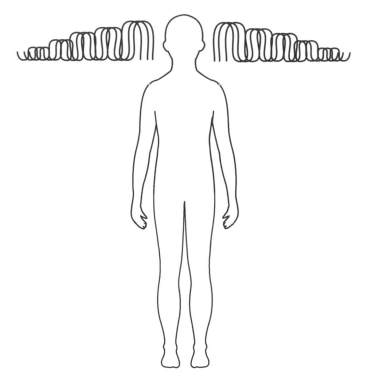

Figure 7.12. PTSD head

Concussions

Concussions are another phenomenon that turn up in both the sixth and seventh chakras. It is contraindicated to work on fresh concussions due to the swelling in the brain, but concussions that are several months old can be worked on gently, and those older than a year can be worked on more deeply. I have found concussions far out on the timeline, from early childhood accidents, that still affect the person as an adult, causing issues such as memory problems, cognitive challenges, and structural imbalances. Athletes who have experienced multiple concussions, especially ones where they have lost consciousness, often develop patterns of behavior that involve extreme frustration over situations that they cannot control, and they experience rage episodes as a result. Biofield Tuning can locate and disrupt this pattern, resulting in calmer, clearer thinking and feeling in people who have suffered from this pattern.

Third Eye Intuition and Perception

The third eye refers to the pineal gland, which, like the regular eyes, has rods and cones for receiving light. My sense is that the light frequencies it perceives are from the higher wavelength of energy—aetheric energy—that passes through the solid bone of the skull and is seen by the mind's eye. People with developed third eyes may see energy patterns in people's bodies, be able to do intuitive medical diagnoses, or see colors in people's energy fields.

The back of the third eye chakra can relate to "things in the back of one's head" (i.e., unfinished projects, unresolved issues, things we may be trying to put behind us but can't due to a lack of resolution). Because this is the area in the brain where ocular function resides, when people have a tendency toward eye strain or headaches behind the eyes, you may find static in this area.

CROWN CHAKRA →← SEVENTH PLEXUS

Color: White or purple
Governs: Brain, relationship with time, relationship with the
    Divine
Relates to: Higher thinking, spatial intelligence, music
Left-side imbalance: Undefined
Right-side imbalance: Undefined
Overall low energy: Difficulty focusing, overwhelmed
    by life, often a consequence of too much time indoors,
    especially under fluorescent lights
Healthy/balanced: Right relationship with time and the
    Divine, aided by plenty of time outdoors

Just like the sides of the feet, I have been unable to specifically determine what the information encoded on either side of the crown chakra

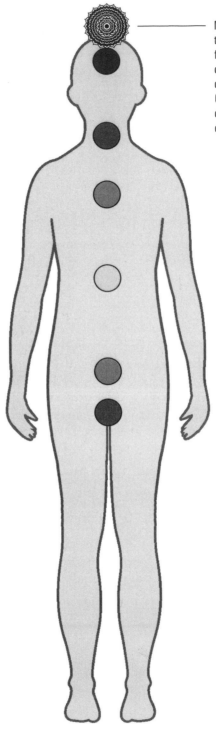

Not enough time; disconnect from nature; difficulty focusing; overwhelmed by life (applies to the area over the top of the crown chakra)

Figure 7.13. Crown Chakra—Seventh Plexus
Higher thinking, spatial intelligence, music

relates to. One of the things that may come up in the crown chakra is higher-order thinking, including math and music. My form of dyslexia makes those particular areas very challenging for me, and this may account for why I don't have a clear understanding of what might be stored on the sides of the crown chakra. Sometimes I find head injuries or concussions here, in addition to the ones I might find in the sixth chakra, especially if it involved a blow to the top of the head. But if there is an emotional or mental story storage system on either side of this chakra (and I would imagine there must be), I haven't figured it out yet. I have figured some other things out about this chakra, though.

If energy is running fast at the crown, it can relate to being in *wrong relationship with time*. And what I mean by the relationship with time is this: our inner experience of our to-do list. At first when I discovered this relationship with time in the crown chakra, I was confused. The crown chakra is generally perceived as relating to our relationship with the Divine. Why would our relationship with the Divine and our relationship with time show up in the same place?

We've all had the experience of feeling as if we don't have enough time to do everything that needs to be done—we run around like a chicken with its head cut off, feeling stressed and pressured and ungrounded. So this was confusing to me until I came across the following quote: "Faith is knowing you have enough time to do everything you have to do." Here was faith and time in the same equation! Suddenly, I saw that we can only be in relationship with the Divine if we are fully in the present. If we are not in right relationship with time, not in the groove, we are not in right relationship with life itself. And when we are in right relationship with time, everything flows nicely; we have many synchronistic encounters and are generally able to maintain a peaceable countenance.

Exercise: If you find yourself becoming tense or upset and believing you don't have enough time, take some things off your to-do list. You are trying to do too much.

I have observed that people who work under fluorescent lights tend to have disturbances in the crown chakra, whereas people who are outside a lot do not. I think one of the best things you can do for your energetic health is to get outside as often as you can, ideally barefoot.

I have observed these patterns in the biofield anatomy of hundreds of individuals. These tendencies are by no means carved in stone, and while they provide a useful guidepost, I absolutely invite you to listen to your own mail slot when you get started using the forks, which we will learn how to do in the next chapter.

8

GETTING STARTED WITH THE FORKS

Choosing Your Forks and Putting Them to Use

The quieter you become, the more you can hear.

RAM DASS

Have you ever gotten a "bad vibe" from someone? And have you ever used the power of music to shift your mood?

If you answered yes to both of those questions, great! You've got what it takes to be a Biofield Tuning practitioner—or really, a sound or music therapist of any kind. You've felt people's vibes, which means that you're attuned to your own ability to read the language of vibration, and you're aware of the power of sound to shift your energy and state of mind.

The ability to sense vibration is a biological reality of your body, and it's the main skill involved in the practice of Biofield Tuning. It's not just your ears that are picking up information that you hear from the forks. On a much more fundamental level it's your body that is sensing the vibrations in the field.

In Biofield Tuning, tuning forks are used in both a diagnostic and a therapeutic manner. The tuning forks act like an invisible ink decoder revealing the exact vibrations that are coming off people. We use the forks to detect areas of resistance, distortion, and noise in the biofield—and to correct them. When we work with the forks we are working with the basic physics principles of resonance and entrainment.

The tuning forks will initially resonate with whatever distortion is present. Let's say it's anxiety: the tuning fork will resonate with the frequency of anxiety in the person's energy field. You can hear it and feel it. But then, the fork will begin to produce a coherent signal. When maintained for a sufficient length of time, what the introduction of this coherent sonic input does is entrain the body into a more coherent expression.

By staying with the fork in these places of noise and resistance, the body becomes aware of its own noise and autocorrects itself. That sense of static, resistance, and distortion will actually resolve. The fork also acts as a metronome, helping the body find its right rhythm. If something is moving too fast, the frequency of the fork helps slow it down. If something is moving too slow, it helps speed it up.

While the basic method is very simple, Biofield Tuning, as a full practice, uses a very specific protocol that's more complex than what can be taught in a book. While the best way to learn is hands-on from an experienced practitioner and teacher, it's possible to begin exploring the method on your own. With the instructions provided in this chapter, you'll have enough information to start using the forks on yourself and others. If you're a massage therapist or chiropractor or any other kind of wellness provider, this chapter will give you enough information to begin integrating tuning forks into your practice.

This overview will provide you with a few basic techniques to start using the forks on yourself or others. If you'd like to explore further, I have several video demos on YouTube, as well as instructional videos available for purchase at www.biofieldtuning.com. If you're interested in becoming a certified practitioner, the first step is our Foundations training programs, which are offered throughout the year both online and in person. You can find more information, dates, and locations for our trainings on the Biofield Tuning website.

In this chapter we'll walk through the basics of choosing and activating the forks; preparing yourself for a session; the process of combing the field (the basic technique in Biofield Tuning) and making an adjustment; and aftercare for both the client and the practitioner. We'll also talk about what to expect as you're learning the language of vibration.

This chapter has been revised and updated for the second edition of Tuning the Human Biofield. Since I picked up my first set of forks back in 1996, the process of Biofield Tuning has been continuously evolving, and it will continue to evolve. Over the years I have greatly simplified and streamlined the basic process while expanding its range of applications and finding new ways to work with the body. With every new client, student, practitioner, and session, the work deepens and expands as we learn more about the human biofield and how it responds to coherent sound.

CHOOSING AND ACTIVATING YOUR FORKS

There is a wide range in the quality of tuning forks available, and this will greatly affect the work you do.

Aluminum forks are preferable to steel forks, as they produce overtones, and overtones are what we are working with and listening for in Biofield Tuning. Machined forks are also preferable to molded forks. Machined forks are cut from a blank, while molded forks are created by pouring hot metal into a mold. I have found the quality of molded forks to be so far inferior to the machined forks that they are, for me, unusable. Medivibe, Omnivos, and Biosonics are all good American-made forks. Having used them all, the Medivibe forks seem to be best suited to Biofield Tuning. My own specialized line of tuning forks are also available in the store on the Biofield Tuning website.

For many years I used the nine-piece unweighted standard Solfeggio set. Over time I have greatly simplified the process I use and teach, such that four forks are sufficient to do a full Biofield Tuning session. My "workhorse" fork is the 174-Hz (Hertz) fork. This fork is what you can use very easily for what I call "field combing." I've tried many, many different frequencies in the field, and there's something about this particular frequency that is ideal for this work. It's in a good range that gives me more feedback than other frequencies. I've settled on the 174-Hz fork as my primary tool because it gives me very useful feedback with the range of audible overtones it emits. This is feedback that you will learn to recognize over time as you engage in the work.

Unlike other healing modalities that use tuning forks, in Biofield Tuning we're not working with the premise that you need to use specific frequencies to tune specific chakras or organs. What we do, instead, is find resistance in the field and simply stay there with a coherent sonic input. It's much more about biofeedback. We're allowing the body to hear its own noise and then self-correct. You can pretty much use any tuning fork in this process. Your body knows its own coherent expressions (what I call its "factory settings"), and it just needs to be able to hear itself rather than any other specific frequency to be able to get back to its natural harmony. I have found it unnecessary to use all kinds of different sounds to remind the body which energy centers need to be resonating at which frequency—it already knows.

In addition to the 174 Hz, I will bring in a 528-Hz fork (or alternately, a 417 Hz), typically after using the 174-Hz fork, as a way to lighten and clarify the tone of the body. After you go through the field with the 174, it's a good idea to follow up with another pass through with one of these higher-frequency forks. The 528- and the 417-Hz forks can be used pretty much interchangeably in the field, or they can be used together on either side of the head to create a binaural beat of 111 Hz, stimulating the production of gamma waves in the brain. When it encounters a pocket of tension, the 528 sometimes emits a screechy sound. I offer the 417 as an alternative in these cases because it doesn't have this quality and it's a little easier on the ears. However, it doesn't have the crystalline brilliance that the 528 has. I recommend experimenting with both and finding your own preference.

The other two forks in our Biofield Tuning toolkit are a pair of weighted forks. What I mean by "weighted" is that they have metal disks attached to the ends of each tine. This makes the vibration go on longer and stronger, making them more beneficial for work in which the handle of the fork is placed directly on the body. What I use and recommend in the way of weighted forks are the 62.64-Hz and 54.81-Hz varieties that we sell at the Biofield Tuning store on our website. These two weighted forks, when combined, create the Schumann resonance (7.83 Hz), as discussed in chapter 5. They comprise the 7th and 8th harmonic of this important frequency of the Earth's ionospheric cavity. They can be used together to create the binaural beat of 7.83 Hz, which can be applied to the body via the handles or listened to in either ear. Placing one handle of each fork on either side of the head and introducing the Schumann resonance can be very soothing for an overactive mind. The frequency of 7.83 Hz is also on the alpha-theta brainwave cusp, which is the state of dreams, REM sleep, and deep meditative states.

If you only want to start with one fork, I recommend the Sonic Slider (93.96 Hz). This is a weighted fork with an extralong handle; it is the 12th harmonic of the Schumann resonance (7.83 x 12), a very pleasing vibration, and can be used on the body and in the field, on yourself as well as on others. Again, I invite you to try the different frequencies and do your own experimenting with whichever forks you would like to use.

Sandpaper is a helpful analogy for understanding the unique effects of the different tuning forks. If we look at tuning forks like grits of sandpaper when we're working through the field, the 174-Hz fork is akin to a medium-grit sandpaper, suitable for most uses. The lower frequency weighted forks are like a coarse-grit sandpaper, while the higher frequencies, like the 528 and 417, are more of a fine grit, best for polishing and refining, as opposed to broad-strokes work. They all work well for their specific applications—it just depends on what you're trying to do.

The unweighted forks are better suited for the field than the body itself, as the biofield is composed of a more subtle energy that requires a finer grit. When used on the physical body, the unweighted forks won't give you much vibration. They're designed for the vibration to come out from the tops of the tines and make sound. A weighted fork, which creates less sound and a coarser vibration, is optimum for sending vibrations more deeply into the body.

I have experimented with many ways of activating the unweighted forks and found that the best thing to use is a hockey puck. Most tuning fork sets come with a rubber mallet or a little triangular striker, and I have found them both to be frustrating and inadequate. Canadian hockey pucks, which are made from vulcanized rubber, are the best, I've found. Other pucks seem to have plastic in them, which produces an unpleasant sound.

To activate an unweighted fork, you'll want to hold the puck like a frisbee, with half of the puck exposed and your thumb on top and other four fingers wrapped around the bottom. Hold the puck securely, exposing enough of the surface so as not to hit your hand with the fork. Hold the handle of the fork gently but firmly in your dominant hand and be sure to not grip the tines of the fork, as this dampens the sound production. Strike the outer edge of the fork, around 1.5 to 2 inches down from the top, against the top edge of the puck in a flicking motion, making sure the tine of the fork is flush with the edge of the puck. Strike firmly and quickly. Before you reactivate the fork, stop the vibration of both tines. If this seems confusing, you can watch Biofield Tuning instructor Michele Kasper do a detailed visual instruction at our YouTube channel.

To activate a weighted fork, grip the fork by the handle, holding the bottom part of the tines underneath the U (holding the fork above the U will diminish the vibration). You can activate the fork by striking the round barrel at the end of the tine gently against your hip, knee, the heel of your palm, or the puck. You don't need to hit the fork hard; it is designed to be activated with just a tap. Try to avoid clanging the tines. It's okay if the fork clangs, but a nonclanging, just-right activation will vibrate longer and stronger. Make sure the weighted forks are blurry when you look at them to be confident you've gotten a good activation. If you're activating both weighted forks at the same time, strike one after the other on either side of the body (usually the hips or knees). Do not hit yourself with both forks at the same time. Another option we recently introduced at the Biofield Tuning store is a green rubber tabletop activator that is great for weighted forks. You can also hold this in your hand, and it can make the process a lot easier.

Activating forks can be surprisingly awkward at first! Keep at it and it will become second nature.

USING THE FORKS ON YOURSELF

Before using the forks on others, spend some time playing with them yourself. Practice activating them; listen to each tone and notice how each one makes you feel. Try listening to two at a time (the 417 and 528 forks combine to make a binaural beat of 111 Hz, within the gamma brain-wave range of focus and productivity). Place the handle of each of the weighted forks on your body—soft tissue, bony spots, different points on your face, hands, and feet—and pay attention to your inner space while you experience the vibration. How does the sound or vibration inspire your body to move, open, stretch, lengthen, or soften?

If you're ready to go a little deeper, try projecting a hologram of yourself onto a treatment table or bed, and then tuning your hologram. It's more straightforward than it sounds. Simply use your imagination and intention to project a representation of yourself onto a mat, massage table, or whatever surface you'd work with a client on. Some people find it helpful to place stones or crystals at the energy centers or to use other contextualizing details. You can also use some kind of stand-in to hold the space of the hologram you're projecting. (I have a skeleton named Mr. Bones in my office that I occasionally use in group sessions.) Because I like to keep things simple and efficient, my preferred method is to just use my intention and declare, "This is my hologram."

Earlier in my practice I had many students ask me if it was possible to do a tuning on yourself, and I always said no. I was of the mind that what makes the process so effective is the triangulation in witnessing between the therapist, the client, and the forks, which act as a relatively objective way of revealing what is presenting in the client's energy field. As a therapist, a huge part of my role is to witness, with my client, the record of past experiences that have not yet been fully processed. It's the witnessing and validation and presence with the person's suffering that supports the healing process. I assumed back then that you don't have that kind of witnessing when you're working on yourself.

Several years later I changed my tune on this matter. I was working in a Faraday cage (an enclosed room that's shielded from electromagnetic fields) with Biofield Tuning teacher and research scientist Jessica Luibrand, as an experiment to see if I could effectively conduct a group tuning in that setting. As a control, I decided to first do a session on my own hologram to try out the Faraday cage before I did a session for three hundred people. I was working on myself, and I hit an obstacle around self-love on the right side of my heart, in an area corresponding to a trauma I experienced between the ages of three and four. In that moment of encountering a painful aspect of this wound that I had never encountered before, I realized that I was being witnessed. I felt that I was being witnessed by the universe, nature, the whole, God—whatever you want to call it.

It was a very powerful experience. It is now my belief that no matter what, we are being witnessed. There is an objective presence that is the universe in its totality that is always witnessing us, so the observer is still there. That can be "spiritual," but it doesn't have to be. For me it was about realizing that I'm just one cell in the organism of creation.

When you are practicing on yourself, remember that this is a process of exploration. It's all right if you don't know what to do. Just jump in and be willing to play and be curious. You're not going to mess up if you work on your own hologram. Do be mindful, however, that the work can run deep. If some heavier inputs come up, a self-session could trigger mild fatigue and emotional release, but that's usually about the extent of it. I once gave myself a tuning in a hotel room in San Diego and was caught off-guard when I encountered some emotions and thought patterns relating to poverty in my mother's lineage. I actually knocked myself out as a result of the session and ended up taking a four-hour nap, but then I felt a sense of greater lightness and clarity after I got up. The work can be easy-peasy, but it can also be very powerful. Be open to whatever outcome arises.

Another way to use forks on yourself is the way the Sonic Slider is designed to be used. The Sonic Slider has an extralong handle that you can activate and then slide along the body in firm strokes, toward the heart. It's similar to the idea of dry brushing, if you have ever done that, except with a vibrating tuning fork instead of a brush.

When I first started using the Sonic Slider on my body in this way I was surprised and delighted to suddenly drop fifteen pounds in just five weeks! Please note that this is not everyone's outcome from using this tool. I am somewhat of an outlier, although there are others who have also had dramatic outcomes. However, most outcomes are more moderate and some bodies don't shrink an ounce. We are each unique. Users report a wide variety of other benefits, including more toned muscles, firmer skin, improved digestion, increased energy, reduced pain and inflammation, better sleep, and interestingly, things like more synchronicities and an improved sense of well-being.

Recently I created another set of weighted forks, also with long handles, based on the Fibonacci sequence. These forks are 89 Hz and 144 Hz, the 11th and 12th positions in the sequence, and together they create the information of Phi, or the Golden Ratio. Whereas the Schumann forks are designed to inform our electromagnetic bodies, the Fibonacci forks are designed to inform our "aetheric template" (i.e., the underlying geometric framework of our bodies). These forks can be used interchangeably with any of the weighted forks, including sliding them on the body. You can learn more about all the forks at www.biofieldtuning.com.

LEARNING THE LANGUAGE OF VIBRATION

A regular participant in my group sessions said to me once, "Your tuning fork is like a magic wand, only better, because it speaks and you know what it's saying." It's not just me, though, as all tuners develop this skill in time.

There is valuable information in the changing tone of the fork as it passes through the person's field. The fork reveals the emotions, stories, and blocks present in the field. With practice you will eventually find that you're able to translate what the forks are saying. For me, it was like teaching myself Braille. Every new vibration I identified and decoded was like adding a new word to my vocabulary.

We really are learning a new language here. Like French or Swahili or any other language, it can be learned by anyone with persistence and a willingness to devote some time and energy to the undertaking. In the beginning of the evolution of this work, there was a perception that I had some kind of unique ability to discern very subtle information—that I could hear and feel and sense things that others do not or cannot sense. Back in 2010, when I was about to start my first class, one of my brothers said to me, "Can what you do be taught?" I said, "I don't know, but I'm going to find out." And what I found out is that anyone can learn this, and the more they stick with it, the more they will experience. In short, anyone can learn this new language over time.

A student reported to me about her first practice body after taking the Foundations class: "The session was remarkable in that I identified the exact years of trauma three times, one of them being in utero. I thought that would take many, many hours of practice. The practice body was stunned at the experience and has already booked two more sessions. This is a person I did not know before this week, so I really knew nothing about her." These kinds of experiences are not uncommon. Thousands of students have gone through our trainings and have had similar observations and experiences using the forks in the field.

This work is not about being psychic or clairvoyant or clairaudient. You're just using your ordinary senses of hearing, feeling, and seeing to interpret the wave forms that you're encountering. When I am teaching students how to use the tuning forks, they tend to be universally surprised and delighted when they encounter resistance in a person's field, meaning they can find the stuck energy and then move it. There is an actual magnetic interaction going on here. It doesn't matter if you think you have no idea what's going on. If you move the fork slowly through the field, it's going to stop on its own when it hits something. The fork will be magnetically grabbed by an energetic tangle. It will feel like physical "stuff," or it could show up as a rush of heat in your body, or you might suddenly stop breathing or feel the fork get jumpy. There's valuable information in all of your body's natural responses.

PREPARING FOR THE SESSION

Centering and Grounding

Before a session take a moment to center yourself and ground your energy. This will help you to come fully into the present moment, let go of any expectations or preconceptions, and just pay attention to the feedback from all of your senses.

Whenever you work with tuning forks, make sure you're in bare feet or socks. Start by grounding yourself, becoming aware of the electromagnetic exchange between you and the surface of the Earth. You are like a lightning rod, and you want the energy that moves through you to be free to release into the ground instead of getting stuck in your body. This is beneficial for both you and the client.

It can be helpful to develop some kind of grounding routine to anchor yourself before starting your sessions. You can visualize dropping a grounding cord from your root chakra down into the center of the Earth, or take a few moments to practice what in Biofield Tuning we call a "centering and grounding breath." (Ideally, do both.) Practicing this breath is very simple. Breathe into your belly, into the area behind and below your navel. As you take a few breaths there, start to relax the area around your tailbone. On your next breath into your belly, use your intention and attention to exhale the energy down and out your tailbone, or down your legs and out the bottoms of your feet. We're centering by bringing our breath deep into the belly, and we ground by consciously sending that energy down and out of the system.

This is a wonderful exercise to practice not only before a session, but whenever you encounter resistance and charge in your field or in the other person's field. Throughout the session, effective grounding is the most useful way to ensure that you do not hold on to the energy of your experience with the other person. Be sure you breathe deeply and maintain a conscious connection to Earth (ground) at all times. This will enable you to allow whatever challenging vibrations you encounter to pass right through you.

Sometimes you may find you have to do what I call "breathing like a boss." If you get into something intense, it can feel overwhelming, and you absolutely do not want your own stuff triggered while you are working with others. That is why we need to practice what we call hollow bone.

Cultivating the Inner State of Hollow Bone

Hollow bone is the inner state that the practitioner should maintain while working on another person. This means exactly what it sounds like: you use a clear intention to remove yourself and your "stuff" to whatever degree is possible from the equation, neutralizing and settling your own emotional state. Adopting this state will enhance the effectiveness of the session by eliminating any personal influence over your perceptions. An energy-sensitive student in my first class remarked that when she was lying on the table with her eyes closed, she could feel each person's energy when they worked on her, but could not feel my energy at all and was only aware of the sound and the feel of the tone produced by the fork while I was working. This is what you want to aim for. A neutral witness, just observing. At the beginning of your practice, this may require some effort, but it gets easier over time. As you become more comfortable and familiar with the hollow bone state, you will be able to perceive the difference between the client's energy and your energy.

A simple exercise to get into hollow bone is to do a quick body scan, starting at your feet and ending at the top of your head. But for this particular body scan, instead of feeling into the different parts of your body as you normally would, focus instead on your bones. Starting from your toes, imagine yourself from a skeletal perspective. As your awareness visits each of your bones, imagine that you are lighting them up, using the light of your consciousness to illuminate your bones. Our bones are piezoelectric—they carry a charge, meaning they have light in them—so as we bring our mind to them, we light them up. Light up all the bones in your whole body, and when you reach all the way up to the crown of your skull, feel the opening of your crown chakra and imagine white light pouring down into your being, splitting off into the colors of the rainbow as it moves through each of your energy centers.

Once you have prepared yourself for the session, set your intention to simply help in whatever way you can, and to do no harm. The homeodynamic intelligence of the body knows exactly what needs to be done and is always working with all available resources to support a state of order, structure, and functionality. You are using the tuning forks to support this process. Stay curious and ask: "What's going on? What wants to happen?"

Whenever I am doing a tuning, I try to be curious, neutral, and open, rather than bringing any specific intentions to it beyond the basic intention to serve. I'm just listening; I'm curious about what's going on and what wants to happen. The body knows better than me (as the practitioner), and even better than the conscious mind. The body knows what's going on and what it needs. I find that it's better to keep our intentions and conscious mind out of the process and to just remain curious and responsive to what's happening in the moment and what you're noticing. As you become more skilled in your practice, there are many different ways to begin to work with the magic of intention, which we explore in our advanced trainings.

For now, focus on cultivating a state of neutrality. Remember that your ability to help others heal has a lot to do with your own state of mind and body. The more clear, coherent, and present you are, the better you can serve others.

Reading the Field

There are many different ways that we receive information from the field. The first thing is to tune in to what you're feeling in the fork. Everyone I've ever taught is able to feel resistance, even if they have a hard time at the very beginning. You hit a certain patch in the field and suddenly it's difficult to move the fork. You've been moving right along, and all of a sudden the fork doesn't want to budge. It starts to feel like you're moving through molasses. You might also notice that the vibration feels different in a certain area. The vibration that the fork is sending into your hand becomes stronger and more intense, or it gets erratic and jumpy.

You're also listening to the sound that's being produced by the fork. As you move through the field, the tone and volume of the sound being produced by the fork will change. An area of charged-up energy will produce a louder tone. Sometimes a patch of resistance will generate an audibly distorted or off-pitch sound. Sometimes the sound will be muffled and run out quickly. When you're starting out, it's the change of tone that you want to listen for.

With practice you will begin to recognize the high-pitched sound of alarm and the low drone of depression. But don't expect to hear the difference right away. People often get impatient about not being able to hear the distinctions in the sounds right off the bat, but the fact of the matter is that it takes time to learn this language of vibration, just like it takes time to learn any language. Then suddenly you're in a session and you hear something in the forks that sounds just like loneliness. Knowing the timelined structure of the field, you'll be able to tell the person roughly what age you're at. Maybe the person was six years old when their dad left, and that's what you were hearing in the forks. That vibrational feeling manifested into vocabulary is now a part of your language. The next time you encounter it, you don't have to figure it out because you already know what it is. It takes time to parse out the sound of melancholy, overwhelm, rage, or shame. The last emotion I identified was fear, and fear is actually one of the most obvious ones! But I couldn't hear it because I couldn't recognize fear in myself, so I couldn't recognize it in anyone else. Your own degree of emotional awareness and intelligence is going to inform the subtleties and nuances that you can perceive, resonate with, and identify.

What you're hearing or not hearing is only one part of the equation. I have found that most people's primary sensory pathway, especially when they're just starting out, is not through their ears. Around 60 percent of the people in my classes are more kinesthetic than they are auditory, meaning they are more likely to feel through their fingertips when the fork gets more "vibrate-y" (in the words of my son Cassidy), as opposed to the 30 percent who primarily hear the change in tone. Around 10 percent of students struggle to hear or feel in the very beginning, but always seem to stop when they hit resistance regardless. We have found that hearing loss is not a barrier to learning this modality because there are many alternate and effective pathways of receiving information.

Depending on whether you tend to be more kinesthetic, auditory, or empathic/intuitive, you'll receive the information in different ways. Each person will come at it from their own angle, and it's all valid. Highly sensitive people often have clear information dropping in through their mail slot about what's going on right off the bat. They'll see images or be able to correctly describe what's there based on their sense of inner knowing. For those who are more kinesthetic, the information will show up as bodily responses. When you enter the field, you go into a state of resonance with the person you're working on; your energy system mirrors and harmonizes with theirs.

I was working on a friend of mine who was having reproductive health issues concentrated around her uterus and ovaries. While I was working on her I felt this intense pain in my pancreas. Even though her symptoms were in her reproductive areas, my pancreas was hurting like crazy. I reached out my hand to touch her pancreas, and it was hard as a rock. What we discovered in that session was that her pancreas had been playing a major role in her symptoms. I never would have thought to go there if it hadn't been for my own pain. There's nothing woo-woo about this. It's simple physics—resonance—no different from when you pluck one string on an instrument and the other strings tuned the same way on nearby instruments vibrate.

It's important to notice what's going on in your body. Are you feeling anxious all of a sudden? Did your temperature change? Are you feeling tension in your chest or stomach? Are you holding your breath? New practitioners often experience these kinds of physical responses and think that it's just them, but it's not just you! It's your body resonating with a part of the field that's holding information about anxiety.

Distinguishing Open vs. Closed Tone

In Biofield Tuning there is a phenomenon we call "open tone versus closed tone." While you are combing you always want to work with an open tone. An open tone sounds like a note sung with your mouth open—clear, resonant, and full-bodied. A closed tone sounds like a note sung with your mouth closed—muffled, dull, and diminished. Oftentimes when someone first gets their hand on a fork, their body will absorb or seemingly "suck up" the sound, resulting in a closed tone wherever they hold it. After a short time, however, this no longer happens because we reflect rather than absorb the sound. Also, you are nervous or have some doubt about your ability to use the forks, their energy can create a static and closed tone.

If you start with an open tone and then it closes, it means that you've gone past the edge into the bulk of what you're moving. If this happens, go back to the edge of the field, find the open tone, and move in again until you hit resistance.

Most importantly: let the fork respond to what is present and trust your senses. Doubt and fear create static that makes this process more difficult than it needs to be. Try to keep your head out of it. Remain open and curious! Trust yourself!

Please note: The actual Biofield Tuning process that we teach in class is more complex than can be covered in this chapter. What I am sharing here is the premise of what I call an adjustment—combing through the field, picking up stuck energy, and returning it to the midline of the body, integrating it and focusing it. This basic idea can be incorporated with different tools as well—hands, singing bowls, or whatever you can think of. Please also note that only certified practitioners are able to call what they do Biofield Tuning, but you are welcome to use the term *sound balancing.*

WORKING IN THE FIELD

Combing

Before you start working on someone, it's important to let them know that their job is to pay attention to how they are feeling while you are working, and also to breathe. Teach them the same centering and grounding breath described above. Sometimes people are very sensitive and can feel things going on right away, and sometimes they might feel nothing at all—either way is okay. Have them take their shoes off and visualize being connected to Earth through their breath. A receiver can be sitting in a chair, or lying on a bed, couch, or treatment table.

As you approach the field, hold the unweighted fork with a relaxed grip, making sure you are not grasping the tines. The more relaxed you are, the more you will hear, feel, and sense. You can, however, rest your thumb gently on the base of the tines. Begin by holding the fork perpendicular to the floor and in line with the body, starting five to six feet from the side of the body. Make sure that your body is open to the client, with your palm facing their body (as opposed to the back of your hand). (See figure 8.1 on page 188.)

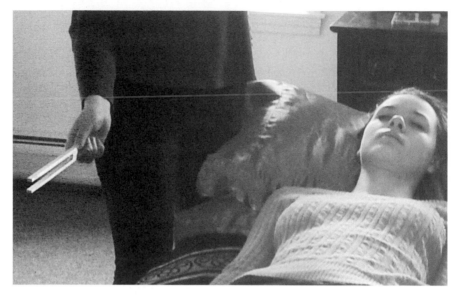

Figure 8.1. Photo showing fork position for combing

There are many ways to approach figuring out where exactly to work. You can start wherever there is pain and work that part of the field; you can always work on the feet because in Biofield Tuning, just like in reflexology, we can find information about the whole body through the feet. Or you can use a pendulum over the body, asking it to inform you where the best angle of approach is.

In the early days of my practice I used to go all the way around the body, working with each side of each energy center. But over time my pace has slowed down and the work has ended up going deeper instead of wider, to the point where sometimes I can spend an entire hour or more working slowly and deeply in just one energy center. It's okay to do it either way.

Once you have determined which region of the body you are going to comb in toward, start about six feet or so away, then start moving slowly in toward the body with an activated fork. If you go slowly enough you will encounter resistance at some point, generally between five and six feet away from the body. This is the outer boundary of the field. Some people struggle with finding the edge of the field at first.

Don't think about it—just move the fork slowly toward the body and feel into what you sense in your fingertips.

When you encounter resistance, stop. This is the edge you will be working on moving, or combing, back to the neutral midline that runs vertically down the center line of the body. Take a moment to sense into what you see and feel as the sound winds down a bit.

Stop the fork from vibrating by placing it gently against your palm, deactivating both tines, before you strike it again. You want to have a new, distinct tone every time you strike. Keep in mind that this is the rule for unweighted forks; with weighted forks you can strike them repeatedly without stopping them first.

Restrike the fork and return to the place where you found the edge. If there is a lot of resistance and a lot of noise and activity in the overtones, it is usually indicative of a high charge or significant upset. Sometimes these very noisy places need to simply be stayed with awhile before we try to move them. They're what I call "hangout spots." You're holding the fork steady in patches where it's dense or noisy, waiting for that to resolve and then continuing in toward the body. Whenever I teach this, students are always amazed to discover the changing terrain and how diverse the expressions are that the tuning fork produces.

The process of combing uses a very simple method that I call click, drag, and drop. This method is what makes Biofield Tuning so easy to learn. You simply find the edge (click), move the fork in closer to the body (drag), and stop the fork before the sound runs out (drop). Reactivate the fork and "click" where you last "dropped." Be very deliberate in your motions, as if you were moving a physical entity. Make sure that you stay on the outside edge (the side farthest from the body) of whatever spot you are working on. Although it's subtle, you are indeed moving stuff! If you lose the edge and start to feel uncertain of what's going on, stop the fork, restrike it, then go back and move in toward the body until you find the edge again.

It helps to think of the tuning fork as a magnet and the energy you encounter as a pile of metal filings that the magnet can grab and drag around. If you go too quickly, you will leave some behind. If you go too slowly, you're wasting time. One of the arts of this technique that you will learn over time is how quickly or slowly you can move with each energetic encounter and how to work with it with optimum efficiency.

One of the things you do not want to do is what I call *feathering*. This is moving the fork backward, away from the body, and then forward, toward the body, once you have found and are working with the edge of energy. When the fork is on the edge of the energy pocket you are working with, it's as if you are connected to the body; at this point you should maintain a steady, inward pressure. Pulling it back and forth can be very uncomfortable for people who are energy sensitive, as they will experience it as a sense of tugging.

Making the Adjustment and Columning

Repeat this process of click, drag, and drop until you are around ten inches from the body. Here you'll hit what we refer to as the *ten-inch zone*, an area that holds more recent events and appears to have greater density. You may find it harder to get through this area. As one of my students put it, getting through the ten-inch zone may require you to "downshift to second gear." You'll know what I mean when you encounter it. In this area it may be necessary to increase the amount of fork strikes you're using and apply a firm intention to push through the density.

Another feature you may encounter around ten inches off the body is what I call the *ancestral rivers*. These are two currents of energy that run along either side of the body and seem to be a direct link to the DNA information streams of the father on the right side of the body and the mother on the left side. Working with these constructs has shown me that DNA, rather than being a fixed chemistry, is more like a flowing song. It shows up as a bidirectional current, where upstream (above the head) holds the record of our ancestor's experiences, and downstream (below the feet) contains information relating to our descendents. Any work we do on a person will resonate with this unbroken chain of information in both directions. Because of this, many clients claim to have witnessed changes in their relationships with their parents and children as they go through the process of re-tuning their own DNA into a more coherent song.

When you've made it through this area, continue combing until you are four inches away from the body. The four-inch zone is an area that we do not work with in Biofield Tuning, simply because we are not able to. The magnetic field of the body is so dense here that it seems to grab any energy being moved through it, and it's easy to get stuck here if you get too close to the body. So instead, go up and over the four-inch zone to drop the energy you've combed into the corresponding chakra center, or the midline of the body, keeping the fork four inches or so above the surface of the body as you move over it. Think of the chakra as a spinning vortex that will pull this energy in and redistribute it throughout the body where it is needed. It's important to understand that the energy we are putting back in the body is not "bad" or "negative." It is energy that had been trapped in an incoherent pattern in the field and is inherently neutral. It is through this process of accessing frozen energy and returning it to circulation that we raise our overall energy and become stronger and more free.

Keep paying attention to the click, drag, and drop process even as you work your way across the body itself. Energy doesn't get stuck and imbalanced just in the field, but also within the body. If someone has a lot of pain in, say, a shoulder, you really want to be clicking on the loud spots there and also moving those toward the center.

Once you get within range of the midline, it's easy to leave energy behind, gathering up some but not all of it. It's especially easy to leave it around the rim of the chakra, and since it's invisible, it's not so easy to tell what you are doing there. One of the metaphors I use while teaching is this: If you have ever taught a child to sweep the floor, you know that they will tend to leave some dirt behind where you wouldn't. You also know that they are going to leave the line of dirt that happens with the dustpan and broom. Dropping into the chakra is like using a dustpan and broom. It takes a few more sweeps than you might initially think to get it completely cleaned up.

What I call the *adjustment* is when we bring the energy that was previously stuck in the field and deposit it back into the body where it can circulate. The next step is mixing paint, or integrating the energy, which involves holding the fork in place above the chakra for several strikes after you've made the adjustment. Here we are mixing the frequencies to create a consistent tone. We have the frequency that's in the body and then we introduce this new collection of frequencies into that equation, and we let it blend, much like mixing two colors of paint to make a third color.

After you've done a few strikes of the fork directly over the chakra (remembering to stay above the four-inch zone), then you can begin the final motion of columning. Begin by holding the fork close to the body and then rising up toward the ceiling slowly from there. If you go slowly, you may encounter a few places where the fork stops; stay in those places for a moment and then continue with the upward sweeping. You can move upward as far as your hand can reach. Just as with feathering, do not move the fork up and down over the chakra. Start each movement at the bottom, a few inches above the body, and move only upward. Repeat until the fork sounds loud and clear and bright, and you feel energetically released by the body.

When we column, what we're doing is creating a channel of information and energy flow between the physical body and the front edge of the field, moving out to the unified field. This liberates our awareness from what Eckhart Tolle calls our *pain body*—our history, our habitual knee-jerk responses to things—and connects us to the present moment.

If you do one side of the body it's always a good idea to do at least a little bit on the other side as well. You can use a weighted fork (coarse-grit sandpaper) and move slowly through the field in a gentle, bouncing motion to do what we call a skim coat. This is a faster adjustment that follows all the same steps. It's especially important to do both sides when you work on the head. Another very important thing is that when

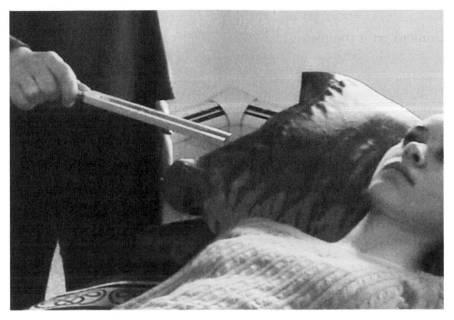

Figure 8.2. Photo showing fork position for columning

you column the crown, you move your fork away from the top of the head—toward the wall if the person is lying down and toward the ceiling if they are sitting up.

That's all there is to it! You can also flip the person over and column the back chakras the same way you column the front, although you do not have to comb the sides if that has already been done on the front. You can then play around with how you want to finish up. In Biofield Tuning we have a closing protocol, but that is a more detailed procedure than we can go into here. Otherwise you can use weighted forks on the body, or I've found that people who practice Reiki can finish with that. I have found it is important to end with the focus at the feet, even if it's just holding them for a moment. If you end at the head, the person can feel ungrounded.

You can also do quick spot treatments instead of working on the whole body, which is useful if you're dealing with a localized ache or pain. These can be done with the person lying on a bed or sitting in a chair. If the person is in a lot of pain, the edge of the pain field may be very far off the body, sometimes six feet or more. It's important to find the edge and work in from there. I keep my forks with me all the time and have on many occasions helped get people out of acute pain in less than twenty minutes.

What to Do If You Get Stuck

What happens if you find yourself in a pocket of turbulence that won't budge? Some areas are just very snarled, and because of this they don't move easily when you encounter them. If you get stuck somewhere—and you will—there are several things you can do to get the energy moving.

Working Directly on the Physical Body

When you're finding it difficult to move the energy in the field, it may be necessary to go to the body. Try using a weighted tuning fork on the body part in question. Tension in the field corresponds with physical tension in the body, and the vibrations produced by weighted forks can interrupt tension patterns in the body. Using two weighted forks of different frequencies next to one another can also be an effective way to interrupt tension patterns in the body.

Using Crystals in the Field

Better yet, you can send the sound through a crystal into the body. Lemurian seed crystals, discussed in chapter 3, seem to be the best tools for the job, but a quartz crystal will also do nicely. Crystals amplify and pulse energy currents if you send a current into one end of the crystal—in this case, by applying the handle of the vibrating (weighted) fork to the flat end. The resulting sound will come out the pointed end in a rhythmic, predictable, amplified pulse. As these sound pulses travel through the body, they dissolve areas of congestion, allowing electricity, blood, and lymph to flow more freely.

When you're first learning to apply sound through a crystal, ask the person you are practicing on if the pressure you are using is too much or not enough. You want it to be firm but not too firm because you are applying the pointed end of the crystal to the body. You may also wish to consider "gem boots" for your forks—little boots that screw onto the base of the handle of weighted tuning forks. However, I prefer working with natural crystals that have points.

While it can be useful to have some knowledge of acupuncture points, trust your magnetic sense of where you see and feel the forks would be useful for applying sound pulses into the body. Usually three or four applications, in a few different spots on the side of the body in the region of the chakra, are sufficient. Almost magically, when you go back to the field after doing some work on the body, you will find the tone has opened up and the energy is moving more easily.

Be sure to keep your crystal clean by washing it in cold water between sessions. When you can, let it rest in the sunshine or moonlight for a day to help clear the energy.

Using the Client's Biological Timeline

Another way to get a spot unstuck is to identify it. For example, if you are on the left side of the third chakra of a forty-five-year-old woman and you encounter resistance around a third of the way to the body from the edge of the field, you can consult figure 3.2 on page 60. As you'll discover, this particular area relates to the relationship with the mother, and that distance from the body suggests a time period around the age of fifteen. You could then tell the person, "According to the map, this area of resistance may have something to do with your relationship with your mother when you were around fifteen, does that make you think of anything?" Some people are very forthcoming and are happy to talk about the fact that they did not get along with their mother at all at that time, whereas others are more private and may not wish to discuss details. It's not necessary for someone to talk about memories or stories in order for the work to be helpful, though.

Naming and Witnessing

One approach we use is to simply ask the person, "What are you noticing?" whenever you get into an area that feels turbulent or off in some way. The client may have discomfort somewhere in their body, a memory arising, or some emotional response. They may not notice anything, and that's okay too. Most people at some point will report that they are getting more relaxed. It's also okay if they don't notice anything. Don't put any pressure on yourself to "heal" someone, just be curious about what you are experiencing and noticing. After all, this work is all about facilitating the body's own self-healing mechanisms.

When I'm doing any Biofield Tuning session, particularly group sessions, I always name what I'm finding. I find that when I name things, especially things that don't seem to be budging even after repeated forays into them, it's brought to light and witnessed. We can examine how it's been affecting us. So part of what we're doing here is just that: bringing these emotions and energetic structures to light. The theory behind why this works involves the power of witnessing. You are acknowledging and validating the person's past experience and the emotions associated with it. Often this bearing witness is all that's required for healing. I will stress here that this part of the job isn't for everyone, and it takes a while for most people to get to the point where they can read the language of vibration confidently.

Know that it is not your job to provide details of what's showing up energetically. It is your job to locate static, resistance, and turbulence in the field and stay with it until it clears. I tend to think of the role more as a technician than a therapist. Also remember that you are not trying to solve the problem. The work of simply bringing the pattern to light and examining it is often sufficient to get it to shift. By simply observing the patterning through the triangulation of (a) the fork, (b) the sound healer, and (c) the client, the charge releases from its frozen position in the field and is returned to the midline of the body, where it can be restored back into circulation.

Moving Energy with the Breath

Bear in mind that the best tool you have for moving energy—aside from the forks—is your own breath.

As practitioners, we're constantly monitoring our breath and using it to discharge energy. A key part of your role as a practitioner is to notice when you're not breathing. Whenever that happens, it's a signal to breathe more deeply and remind your client to keep breathing too.

What you will come to notice is that the moment you hit a patch of heavy distortion, the first thing you're probably going to do is hold your breath. It's that response of sympathetic resonance with what you're finding in the field. You're mirroring the energy that's held in that turbulent moment in the person's history. The first thing we do when we're in an unmanageable situation is hold our breath. When you're seven years old and your alcoholic father is storming through the house, you hold your breath. It's a way to clamp down your emotions and try to disappear. So when you start working on the record of somebody's alcoholic dad, you're probably going to stop breathing. It's going to trigger the same response, both in the client and in the practitioner.

When you get into a tangle like this, you need to breathe, center, and ground. Use your breath to discharge the energy. Breathe into your belly, and take a deep, audible exhalation out of your mouth as you release the energy through your tailbone or feet. This may feel a little strange at first. It took me a while to feel comfortable breathing audibly right next to my clients. But you have to. There's no way around it. When people are struggling in class and feeling like the energy of someone else is too much, I tell them to "breathe like a boss!"

Learning how to breathe, center, and ground is really the simplest exercise I can offer to help you become a better practitioner and to better manage your stress overall. Before every session take a few moments to do the centering and grounding breath. Strive to maintain that deep belly breath as much as possible throughout the session and use it to release any lingering undischarged energy after you've finished.

SONIC DETOX AND AFTERCARE

While for the most part tuning-fork treatments are relaxing and pleasant to receive—most people report feeling lighter, more relaxed, clearer,
and calmer—sometimes the work can create a detox response wherein
the person actually gets worse before they get better. Pain may become
more intense, symptoms may flare up, emotions may surface, several
days of exhaustion may set in, and there may be a sense that the experience made everything worse. However, many years of observation have
showed us beyond a shadow of a doubt that these things are better out
than in!

Some clients have reported:

- Extreme tiredness and exhaustion; needing to rest for a day or
  more. This commonly happens with people who have been "running on empty."
- Heightened emotions, or being very aware of formerly masked or
  buried emotions (overwhelming sadness, crying a lot, being very
  angry or irritable)
- Headaches and/or dizziness
- The release of mucus
- Excessive thirst (it is very important to hydrate well before and
  after tuning)
- In rare instances, skin rashes, fevers, vomiting, loose stools

Generally, these symptoms are an indication of detoxification, and
they pass within a day or two. In these instances I tell clients that if
they do their best not to resist the experience, they will feel better in
one to three days. In rare instances the detox can last for a week or
more, but this is very uncommon.

If a condition persists, it's beneficial for the client to receive a follow-
up session—sooner rather than later. Sometimes people can get stuck in
the unwinding process and need an additional boost to complete the
adjustments. We have observed that conducting sessions in series of

three with a week or so in between is an effective general approach to this work. However, there is no limit to the amount of sessions one can receive, as each one builds on the one before it. Ultimately, there is no end point to healing. I have received over five hundred sessions at this point, and there is always another layer to work through, always more potential to access.

After any session, to support the clearing and integrating process I always recommend lots of water, inside and out. Tell your clients to drink plenty of water and herbal tea. The best thing you can do after a session is to soak in a Epsom salt bath for at least twenty minutes (or even better, go in the ocean if possible). This supports the body in detoxifying or releasing any physical components of the blockages released from the energy field. It's also beneficial to be well hydrated before a session due to the sound-conductive properties of water.

As a practitioner, you will find water can also be beneficial for clearing your own energy after a session. Wash your hands slowly and mindfully while saying with intention, "May anything I picked up here be released into the Earth." If I have a particularly challenging day and have dealt with a lot of trauma, I take a shower when I get home and envision anything that might be sticking to me washing down the drain. For clearing the space and the forks, many people burn sage or palo santo. There are many different tools and rituals for clearing energy. I recommend doing a bit of experimenting to find what works best for you.

CULTIVATING SELF-TRUST

The ultimate key to growing in this work is self-trust. So many of us have been taught to not trust ourselves. Very often when people are learning Biofield Tuning they become aware that they don't trust their own feeling sense. This is what can happen when so many things in our upbringing condition us to defer to external authority instead of listening to and honoring our gut feelings and natural inclinations. I've watched dozens of people in class trying to find the edge of the field. They come in, pause for a moment, and then override and second-guess themselves. They don't trust themselves, and as a result, they don't acknowledge that little imprint they got when they hit the right spot.

Coming back into our own knowing can be a hurdle in this work. The process of working with the forks can help rebuild that trust. The tuning forks can act as training wheels for us to develop our sensory and perceptive abilities. They help us hone our capacity to read the energy around us, which is what we're doing all the time anyway. Remember, what is occurring between the practitioner and client is an actual electromagnetic interaction. The forks simply magnify and amplify the ambient frequencies that we're already feeling. Tuning in to what's happening is simply a matter of listening and trusting your senses.

Not taking ourselves so seriously can help here. At the beginning especially, curiosity is the most important thing. Be curious about what you're noticing and what your client is noticing. This work is a very curious thing! Every session is an adventure. You never know what you're going to find. Even after doing this for twenty-five years, I still never know what's going to happen in any given session. Be willing to play and experiment. Instead of being worried about doing it right and trying to predict or direct what's happening, be more like a little kid, digging and exploring and being curious about what's going on. Every single session is a journey with an unknown destination. We have no idea what's going to happen, and our intention is to stay present in every moment with whatever is arising.

If you would like to watch a demonstration of this process, our Biofield Tuning toolkit contains over two hours of instructional videos that can take you deeper into the process, and if your mail slot is telling you that this is something you would like to offer as a certified professional, check out www.biofieldtuning.com for both online and in-person trainings.

Ultimately, your ability to help others heal has a lot to do with your own state of mind and state of body. The more healthy, coherent, present, and whole you are, the better you can serve others. Fortunately for me, doing this work has taught me so much about the patterns of our subconscious mind, about behaviors that are functional and behaviors that are dysfunctional, and that has really helped me to be a much healthier person myself.

In the following chapter I share some of the most valuable insights I have gained in the hope that they will help you, too, become healthier.

9

BIOFIELD ANATOMY WISDOM

Learning Self-Care—Saying No,
Cultivating Neutrality, and Using
Love as the Ultimate Healing Tool

You have a great body. It is an intricate piece of technology and a sophisticated super-computer. It runs on peanuts and even regenerates itself. Your relationship with your body is one of the most important relationships you'll ever have. And since repairs are expensive and spare parts are hard to come by, it pays to make that relationship good.

STEVE GOODIER

Flip the spin is the name I give for a very simple exercise to help sensitive people deal with "bad vibes" from others or from their environment. I've experimented with different techniques over the years to deal with this issue, and this one seems to be the easiest and the most effective. *Flip the spin* is a metaphor based on the notion that what we call *negative energy* spirals toward us in a direction that causes us to feel worn out, run down, or sapped when we are exposed to it. We may also become sad, angry, or frustrated or feel somehow responsible for this negative energy or a variety of other nonbeneficial feeling states.

When you find yourself in the path of this energy, whether by choice—as in being there for a friend in crisis—or by circumstance, instead of resisting it or trying to erect a barrier to it (very challenging to do, in my experience) you simply "catch it" with the energy of your solar plexus, allowing yourself to feel it for a moment, to empathize with it, and with a clear intent, gently flick it to get it to spin the other way, sending it back to the other person with a positive spin and the feeling of compassion. It's that simple.

When we are really centered and grounded, we can radiate compassion continuously, which is a really nice state to maintain if you can. This is the essence of "lightworking" or spiritual alchemy—turning energetic lead into gold, or heavy, negative energies into light, positive ones. The more you practice it, the easier and more automatic it becomes. People I have shared this exercise with routinely report being amazed at how simple and effective it is.

SAYING NO

One of the things I have observed in this work is the tendency of so many people to say yes when what they really want or even need to say is no. I came to realize how often I did this in my own life. I had been raised by a stay-at-home mom who waited on all of us hand and foot. She fed us three meals a day and did laundry and housekeeping without ever asking for help, and even though we had chores, she took care of most everything. She never took days off, but every once in a while, maybe once every two or three months, she would have to lie down on the couch for a whole day with a migraine, which seemed to be the only way she could justify taking some downtime.

We tend to parent the way we were parented, and I fell into very similar habits as those of my mother (minus the migraines). This worked well for a time, but when I started undergraduate school and was taking eighteen credits as well as seeing clients, it all became a bit too much. I'll never forget the first time I realized that I was simply too exhausted to cook dinner and that I really just needed to go to bed. My husband is a carpenter and was working long days doing physical labor. He had gotten accustomed to coming home spent and was grateful to have a meal on the table. My boys were eight and eleven at the time, and they too were quite accustomed to Mom taking care of everything. On this particular evening I announced to them that I was not cooking dinner, they could fend for themselves, and I went to bed, pulling the covers up over my head, wracked with guilt for saying no.

Since that time I have become much, much better at saying no and taking care of myself when I need to. I've trained my husband and my boys how to make a few different meals (or just get takeout), and I no longer feel the least bit guilty when I need to put my own needs first. Cassidy even said to me the other day, "Mom, if you don't feel like cooking dinner, then just don't. We'll figure it out."

Obviously, as a parent, there are times when you simply can't put your own needs first, especially when your children are very young—which leads us to the next topic:

ASKING FOR HELP

As someone who was born and raised in New England, and having lived in Vermont for the past eleven years, I am very accustomed to the tradition of the self-sufficient individual. New Englanders—and it seems Vermonters in particular—place a high premium on being self-sufficient and not wanting or needing help from others. The irony is that these folks are the first to show up to help others and even thrive on being able to do so.

I had a client who was a giver by nature express to me his sentiment that "whoever gives the most in a relationship wins." I pointed out to him that this was actually a selfish attitude because it made him the winner and didn't give the other person the opportunity to feel the good feelings associated with giving. He was surprised to hear that, as he had not considered this perspective before.

Gracious receiving gives dignity to the act of giving. Being willing to receive help and support allows others to enjoy giving help and support. The fact of the matter is that sometimes we need help, when we are faced with a task that is too big, too overwhelming, too much to do ourselves. It's important to learn to recognize these times—before you throw your back out moving the couch by yourself, or scream at your kids because you really needed a break, or end up late on a deadline because you didn't recognize or realize that someone else could have helped you with it.

There is a personality type that I call "the good soldier" who carries on valiantly, never saying no to anyone, never asking for help, pushing herself well beyond the limits of her body and mind with regularity. And while this may be admirable, ultimately the body rebels—such a person finds herself exhausted, irritable, prone to infections, unable to sleep well, or self-medicating with food, alcohol, drugs, or shopping. To be truly healthy and to maintain a balanced state, it is important to learn to recognize when it is appropriate to say no, and when to ask for help.

THE 80 PERCENT SYNDROME

The 80 percent syndrome describes the propensity for starting a project or task and finishing roughly 80 percent of it but then not seeing it through to the very end. These people's lives are littered with unfinished projects (and often frustrated partners). For me it shows up in things like doing the laundry and folding the clothes, but not putting them away, and instead leaving them on top of the dryer or in the basket or on top of the bureau. For men it can show up in unfinished trim work—last bits of painting left undone or project cars or motorcycles that sit incomplete, taking up space in the garage. For artists it can result in unfinished paintings and sculptures; for writers, in abandoned articles and books. I used to do this myself until I started to understand why this occurs.

This syndrome often arises in people who have a lot of stuck energy in their fields regarding issues with one or the other or both parents. Because the third chakra is the chakra of setting goals and achieving them, our energy to complete tasks comes through here, and if a good portion of one's third chakra vital energy is tied up in the past with unresolved hurts, we won't have the gumption or chutzpah to finish our tasks. It simply isn't there to draw on. So if you have an 80 percenter in your life or if you yourself are one, don't hold it against him or her, or if you are such a person, don't beat yourself up. The good news is that tuning forks can be used to find, break up, and reintegrate this stuck energy so that you can go that extra mile to the finish line. And one of the things that I have learned, as a former 80 percenter, is that that extra mile isn't really that hard or that far, and the payoff, the return on the investment of energy in feeling satisfied, far outweighs the small amount of energy required to go the extra distance to completion.

PURPLEWASHING

Purplewashing is my term to describe the tendency people have to gloss over, repress, or deny uncomfortable emotions, usually by "spiritualizing" the situation or by "being nice" about it. I call it *purplewashing* because it's similar to the concept of greenwashing, wherein corporations that are not really environmentally friendly engage in PR practices and advertising to make it seem as if they are by constructing a green veneer over an uglier truth.

Purplewashers skip anger and go right to forgiveness; they skip jealousy and go right to feeling happy for people; they push aside frustration and smile. They tend to label certain emotions as "bad" and unacceptable, and therefore fail to acknowledge them when they arise in the body. I use the color purple because just as green is considered the color of environmentalism, purple is the color of spiritualism, or the higher realms of thinking and being.

An emotion is an electro-chemical event, and any emotion that is repressed or denied is a repression and denial of one's life force. Neurologist Candace Pert has shown that different emotions have different chemical compositions, and when we experience any of these emotions, their vibrational and chemical counterparts are generated and circulate in our body. When an emotion goes unexpressed or unrecognized, the body does not digest or recycle it, it stores it, or as Pert says, "Emotions buried alive never die."[1] Emotions always find a way of expressing themselves. What this means is that the energy of our emotions is always trying to be heard and expressed in some way, like anything buried alive might. If we don't recognize them for what they are and find healthy ways to express them, they will find a way to express themselves anyway—in sickness or disease, tumultuous life situations, or an eventual mental or emotional breakdown.

A purplewasher can tend to have a sweet tooth; instead of really feeling and expressing anger, she instead consoles herself with chocolate or a glass of wine, thereby pacifying herself but not really doing anything about an issue when action of some sort may be indicated. This explains why unexpressed emotions can also express themselves in excess weight. One place in particular where emotional energy can accumulate as fat is at the base of the neck on the back. We've all seen people who have a lump in this area. The way I have come to understand and explain this fatty area is that it is the home of "the gatekeeper." The gatekeeper decides which emotions may pass into the brain and therefore conscious cognition, and which ones are forbidden.

I have definitely done a certain amount of purplewashing in my lifetime. Up until my midtwenties I barely recognized the emotion of anger in myself. I had grown up with a mother who was a feisty Irish redhead. She was calm and loving most of the time, but when she got angry, she got really angry, and she threw things. She once threw an entire table setting of silverware, plates, and glasses at my oldest brother, who was stuck cowering in the corner of the dining room. After my father's stroke I never knew what was going to be flying around the house. So, after bearing witness to these terrifying displays of anger, I decided that "anger is bad," something I didn't want to feel.

I did the same thing with the emotion of fear. I'm not sure of the origin of this pattern in myself, but I became very good at repressing fear, and rarely if ever consciously recognized it in myself. In fact, it was one of the last emotions I learned to recognize when I was creating the biofield anatomy—which in hindsight is sort of odd given that fear is actually one of the easiest emotions to detect due to its pronounced and distinctive pulsing quality. But we can only recognize in another what we recognize in ourselves, and I had done a very good job of purple-washing fear in myself. A week or so after I finally heard it in a client, I was able to perceive it in myself and was quite surprised and even startled by it. At the time I was working part-time as a gardener, and I was sitting, pulling weeds from under the rosebushes, thinking about our current money problems. My husband was considerably overdue on payment for a large job he had completed, and the bills were start-ing to pile up. We still weren't sure when or even if the check was coming, and I had no idea if we were going to be able to navigate much longer. All of a sudden it dawned on me that I was running the fear current. "That's fear!" I exclaimed, both pleased and surprised to recognize it.

Another emotion I have suppressed is jealousy. The first time I ever really felt consciously jealous of someone was when I was in my early twenties, and it felt like poison running through my veins. *This is a very uncomfortable emotion and I don't ever want to feel this way again,* I told myself. And I didn't, for a very long time. But several years ago I was having a session with a shamanic counselor, and we were discuss-ing emotions. "I don't allow myself to feel jealousy," I told her (this was before the insight about purplewashing). And she said, "Oh, that's strange. Why would you want to stop yourself from feeling any of your emotions?" What a good question that was. The best answer I could come up with was that it was unpleasant, uncomfortable, and that I had judged jealousy as "bad" and cast it out of my awareness. Did that mean that I didn't feel jealousy anymore? Or just that I wouldn't let myself feel jealous? How lofty of me, really, to declare myself above jealousy. Do you see the purplewashing here?

Recently, I had the opportunity to experience the feeling of jealousy, to really let it flow through me. It wasn't pleasant, not at all, but I let myself face it squarely, truly feel it. I also talked to a few friends about my experience—how true it is that confession is good for the soul! Feel the feeling, talk about the experience of the feeling, love yourself even though you are experiencing an unpleasant feeling, and it moves along.

If we don't, then the emotions that we deny tend to fester in one way or another.

I had a client who became defensive when I shared with her that she had a lot of stuck energy in the area that I relate to guilt and shame. This person was suffering from an autoimmune disorder that she had been unable to heal. When I told her what I perceived, she insisted that those weren't feelings that she felt, seemingly implying that she knew better than to feel such base emotions (a sentiment I could obviously relate to). Were her suppressed emotions related to the disease? It would certainly seem so.

The bottom line is that as humans, we all experience the full spectrum of emotions, whether we recognize them or not. Unrecognized emotions act subconsciously in our lives according to the law of reciprocal vibration. What we put out, conscious or otherwise, is what we get back.

According to Human Design a synthesis of several ancient systems, including astrology, the I Ching, the Vedic chakra system, and the Kabbalah, our emotions are a sort of navigation system designed to give us feedback about where we are on our path. They nudge us along, away from that which feels unpleasant or is unhealthy, toward that which is pleasant and healthy and appropriate for us. If we continually purplewash, we may see ourself as doing the right thing, but the quality of our life situation will show us what we are repressing.

MANAGING EMOTIONS

Emotional discomfort, when accepted, rises, crests, and falls in a series of waves. Each wave washes a part of us away and deposits treasures we never imagined. Out goes naivete, in comes wisdom; out goes anger, in comes discernment; out goes despair, in comes kindness. No one would call it easy, but the rhythm of emotional pain that we learn to tolerate is natural, constructive, and expansive. . . . The pain leaves you healthier than it found you.

MARTHA BECK

If you are willing to feel your emotions, you need to be able to know how to handle them, and this isn't something we get a lot of guidance on culturally. Mostly we are simply told that they are not okay, and therefore we are expected to repress them in one way or another. But there are a few simple things we can do to deal with our emotions in a healthy way.

One important observation I have made involves the way people refer to their emotional experiences in different languages and cultures. In Germanic languages such as English and German, we refer to emotions in terms of "being" them: *I am angry, I am sad, I am frustrated*. In the Romance languages such as Italian, French, and Spanish, emotions are referred to in terms of "having" them: *I am having anger, I am having sadness, I am having frustration*. If you look at British people and then at Italians, who is freer in terms of their ability to express emotions?

Try this: Say "I am angry." Then say, "I am having anger." What is the difference in your inner experience when you rephrase how you express your emotions? Which way allows you to feel okay about your emotional experience? Everyone I have ever shared this with finds the experience of *having* emotions preferable to *being* the emotion. Not only is it a more comfortable way of expressing the experience, it is more accurate as well. Remember, emotions are like waves: they rise up, peak, and then fall away—if we allow them to. However, there are many ways to arrest the movement of the wave: smoke a cigarette, eat a chocolate bar, pour a drink, have sex, go shopping, take a pill, point a finger at someone else, mindlessly veg out in front of the TV. Advertising provides us with limitless opportunities to avoid our emotions; it even encourages us to avoid our emotions, profiting off our avoidances. And this is quite helpful, because emotions aren't really permissible, especially for men, in our culture. Men are allowed to feel anger and not much else. How many of you heard growing up, "Big boys don't cry" or "Nice girls don't get angry." We have all been very conditioned by our families and by Madison Avenue to not feel and not express those feelings.

The Centers for Disease Control says that 85 percent of all diseases are caused by stress. What is stress? An emotional response to a situation. Which means that 85 percent (perhaps even more) of diseases are caused by unexpressed, unacknowledged emotions. And yet, when you go to a doctor or a hospital, in most cases you are never asked about your life situation. You are examined, tested, poked, and prodded as if your meat machine was something separate from your emotional body.

A while ago a good friend of mine ended up in the emergency room because she was experiencing sudden tightness in her chest, heart palpitations, and extreme difficulty in breathing. She was put through a battery of tests, kept overnight for observation, and then told that there was nothing wrong with her. As it turns out, she had had a very stressful experience, a sort of last straw with her alcoholic husband, and had a massive anxiety attack over it. She was in a mental and emotional crisis that was so extreme that her body went into overload, but not one person at the hospital had asked her about her mental or emotional state.

Such is the state of modern medicine—and one of the reasons why Biofield Tuning is such a helpful and useful practice. In Biofield Tuning the client doesn't even need to be aware of what's going on emotionally, because the pattern of resistance that shows up with the tuning forks illustrates this beautifully.

I have a client who has a low-grade blood disorder and suffers from low energy. In one of his first sessions he had so much frustration present that it felt like it was literally killing him. He was aware that he was frustrated but didn't realize how much upset it was creating in his body until it was reflected back to him, because it was easy for him to hear the tonal quality of the fork and how dissonant it sounded. He went home with a homework assignment: to be mindful of the current of frustration running through his body. Over the course of successive sessions he displayed less and less of this in his field, as he learned to experience less and less frustration with his life situation through mindful awareness.

Emotions run like guardrails down the sides of our energetic bodies. They provide us with a feedback loop to make the adjustments we need to stay on keel. If we get too bogged down in one emotional state—for example, frustration—it drags us out of balance, or to use a boat metaphor, it causes us to tilt to port. In boats, from the back looking forward, the left side of the boat is port and the right side is starboard. Port tilts are expressed in sadness, frustration, disappointment, and stuckness; starboard tilts are anger, overdoing, guilt, shame, and powerlessness. (I also call these the left-hand ditch and the right-hand ditch.) Actually, going too far to either side leads to powerlessness. One woman described the emotions on either side as being like Velcro walls and described herself as being in a Velcro suit, tearing herself off one side she was stuck to, only to be flung over to the other side and get stuck there for a time.

If we can learn to master really feeling our emotions, acknowledging them, allowing them to guide us to make the course corrections that are indicated for smooth sailing, we will be able to travel through life with much greater ease, the wind at our backs, and our balanced prow cutting easily through whatever waters we are navigating at the time.

THE INFLUENCE OF BELIEFS

Everyone has patterns that they act out over and over again. What I have found is that the tracks that get laid down early in life become the grooves we can get stuck in for the rest of our lives. Although an infinite potential exists in every moment, we continue to choose what is familiar to us, what fits in with our beliefs.

Some of the most significant work I have done using Biofield Tuning has been with beliefs that are formed around the crucial age of seven. I have found that this is the age when we begin to think critically about our environment and the people in it. My younger son brought this to my attention one day. At the time he was in the sixth grade, and I was driving him home from school. "By the time you're in second grade," he said, "you've lost that innocence you had in kindergarten."

Before age seven we take everything as it comes, and we also tend to think that we are responsible for everything; it doesn't occur to us that adults could be at fault for anything. Therefore, anything unpleasant in our world must be our fault. But when we reach the age of seven, we can see that others can also be at fault. Prior to that we can form some very powerful self-limiting beliefs that inform the story of our life. These beliefs are very fixed or stuck when I find them at the outer edge of the field, and the energy sunk in them often doesn't move unless the belief is named.

I liken working with these stuck beliefs to digging burdock. If you've ever dug up burdock, you know exactly what I'm talking about. It requires patience and tenacity to dig up burdock root, and it requires patience and tenacity to uproot a very fixed, self-limiting belief. Another metaphor I refer to is the device that an eye doctor uses to assess your vision, which has many different lenses; the doctor flips the lenses around, asking you which one makes you see better. Fixed, limiting beliefs are like lenses that distort our perception of reality. "I always ruin everything." "No one cares about what I have to say." "My needs aren't important." "Men aren't supportive of me." "Women aren't supportive of me." "I don't deserve to be here." "I'm not good at anything." "I will never amount to anything." "I'm not worthy of love, success, or happiness."

Our senses are subjected to somewhere in the vicinity of forty million bytes of information per second, but we can only process forty bytes per second, which means that we screen out an awful lot of information. Generally, we perceive what fits in with our beliefs about what is possible.

Many of us have come across the story of the native people of South America not being able to see the big boats of the Spaniards when they arrived off their shores, even though they were right in front of their eyes. They couldn't conceive of such things, therefore they could not see them. It was only after the shamans saw them and described them that the ordinary folks could finally see them.

I had a somewhat similar experience of imperception in my twenties. When my mom got her cancer diagnosis, I put all of us on a macrobiotic diet, as I had read that it could be helpful in healing cancer.

Macrobiotics is a diet that consists largely of brown rice and vegetables and eliminates sugar, wheat, dairy, and most meat. I had been living on a diet of sugar, wheat, dairy, meat, and coffee up to this point, so this was a radical departure from what I had been eating most of my life. The macrobiotic diet also includes lots of leafy greens such as kale, collards, mustard greens, and the like, things I had never eaten in my entire life (I was an incredibly fussy eater as a kid). I noticed immediately that I was much calmer on the macrobiotic diet, and although it did nothing for my mother, it definitely helped the rest of us deal with her decline more peaceably than we would have otherwise.

One of the things that happened during this time was that my glasses started to bother me. I had been wearing glasses since I was thirteen for a mild case of nearsightedness, and I assumed that my vision must have gotten worse because that is what happens to people as they get older. So I made an appointment with my eye doctor, anticipating the need for a stronger prescription. Much to my surprise, after examining me the doctor said, "Well, the reason your glasses are bothering you is because you don't need them anymore—you have perfect 20/20 vision." When I drove home without my glasses on, I realized, apparently thanks to my better nutrition, that I actually could see everything at a distance, with none of the accustomed blurriness. I needed an authority to tell me I could see better before I could realize that I *was* seeing better, because seeing better did not fit in with my belief of "I am nearsighted and require glasses." This is how so many of us go through our lives—not seeing or perceiving what is right in front of us because we do not believe it is possible.

How many of you have had the experience of having a particular problem for some time, and then discovering that you had what you needed to remedy the situation all along, you just didn't see it?

CULTIVATING NEUTRALITY

Cultivating neutrality is how I describe the process of acquiring equanimity. What I mean by this is a state where you are neither happy nor sad, neither elevated nor depressed, but simply neutral. I think the edict that Americans are entitled to "life, liberty, and the pursuit of happiness" creates a problem that goes largely unexamined in our culture. There is a significant difference between pursuing happiness and simply being happy, and many people get caught up in the pursuit without ever really "catching" happiness. The staggering number of people who are on antidepressants is evidence alone that something is not working.

Often, if people suffer from depression, they feel a lot of pressure to be happy, but the distance between the low of depression and the high of happiness can seem like such a long way to go. Unable to get to happiness or to hold it once they may fleetingly experience it, they slip back down into depression. People try to think positively, only to find themselves completely overrun with negative feelings and self-reproach. They are gripped by the fear that something is going to come along to take away their happiness, and so they have a hard time even letting themselves feel it for fear of losing it.

When we cultivate neutrality, we don't have to worry about any of this. We understand that life is full of ups and downs; good things happen and bad things happen, and that is the nature of life. We allow ourselves to feel all of our emotions as they arise, labeling none of them as "good" or "bad," but simply seeing that they are part of the human experience. We allow them to play out as they need to with a good laugh or a good cry or maybe a brisk walk or some deep housecleaning if we are angry. When we allow our emotions to run their course, without judging them or repressing them or thinking we shouldn't be feeling them, they move on. It's only when we resist them, repress them, or judge them that they tend to stick around and create problems.

Neutrality is the place that we return to once the highs or lows have passed. And in neutrality, there is a certain peace—nowhere to go, nothing to do, nothing to fix, no agenda to push, no ax to grind, nothing to be except simply being present. This is a lovely space, a state of mind where you can enjoy true rest, where there is no charge of happiness to maintain, no charge of sadness to wallow in or seek to escape from, and the place from where we can create our reality.

CREATING YOUR REALITY,
OR THE LAW OF ATTRACTION

My people can have what they say, but my people keep saying what they have.

CHARLES CAPPS,
THE TONGUE: A CREATIVE FORCE

This quote, from the book *The Tongue: A Creative Force,* by Charles Capps, a retired farmer, land developer, and ordained minister, sums up the essence of reality creation, or the power of the word to create one's reality. What it is saying is that the word is creative, and when we repeatedly say things like "I am broke" or "I am stuck" or "I am sick and tired," that is what we are creating. It's not just in what we say, but also in what we feel.

Most people have reality creation backward. They are waiting for outside circumstances to change before they will say "I am rich," "My life is moving along nicely," or "I feel great," and then experience all the associated feelings that go along with that.

Remember, our life situation is an "exploded view" of our bodies and our fields. The body and its field is primary, is creative, and the life situation reflects that, not the other way around. When we keep saying what we have, we are creating more of that. Anything we resist tends to stick around (what you resist, persists) because we are giving it energy. It is only by being willing to cultivate different words and feelings *first,* and then not giving any attention or resistance to what shows up in opposition of that—because those things will continue to show up for a little while until the new pattern kicks in—that the new pattern begins to show up in the life situation.

Imagine what it feels like to be rich, to be successful, to own your own home, to have a new car; now allow yourself to feel those feelings. I recently heard a story about someone who decided to start treating his old car the way he would treat a new car—keeping it clean and clutter-free, inside and out, feeling the feelings he imagined he would feel in a better car—and in a very short time, a nicer, newer car appeared suddenly and serendipitously in this person's life. Your feelings will truly magnetize to you the outer circumstances that reflect those feelings, but there is a time gap in which faith is necessary, and this is where many people give up.

Here is a very simple exercise you can do anytime. Ask yourself, "How am I feeling? How do I want to feel? What needs to happen in order for me to feel that way, that I can control or affect right now?"

We can't simply flush or eliminate feelings from our bodies without first listening to what they are trying to tell us. Remember, they are there as guideposts to keep you on keel, so if you are feeling a strong emotion, there is a message there for you, an indication that you must change course in some way, take some sort of action, communicate something to someone. Not heeding your emotions can lead you into the rough, and not learning to cultivate emotional discipline can keep you in the rough.

YOU ARE WORTHY

When I first started working with tuning forks, I was very surprised to discover that underneath every person's "noise" is a harmonic signal. And when that signal comes through clearly, the person is what I can only describe as "great." I kept coming home and saying to my husband, "That person I worked on today was great!" I kept being somewhat astounded to discover this in virtually everyone.

Reflecting on my surprise made me realize that I had always just assumed, based on what I had been taught, that humans were imperfect, that we were fallen from grace, that we were fatally flawed somehow. Our Christian cosmology, even in our supposedly secular culture, had wormed its way into my brain and formed a subconscious belief that I was a "guilty sinner." Even though I was actually raised in a religion-free home, the ubiquitous story of Adam and Eve and how they blew it—especially her—had apparently shaped my thinking without me realizing it. So here I was, surprised to see that this was not true—that here was the potential of perfect harmony, an aspect of humanness that was not out of sync with the universe, not out of step with nature, but actually quite in sync, beautifully, pleasingly, even jaw-droppingly in sync. I have never worked on anyone who does not have this harmonic potential.

The thing is, most of us associate with what spiritual teacher Eckhart Tolle calls our *pain body*. This is the aspect of the self that has borne all the wounds of one's lifetime—traumas small and large, on every level of being. These can even be inherited traumas that have been vibrationally encoded into our energetic blueprint. Most of us don't believe that clear harmony exists as a potential within each of us, and even if we did, the belief that we are not worthy would get in the way. I have found at the kernel of every dysfunction, at the core of every issue, this belief: *I am not worthy*.

I invite you to see where and how *I'm not worthy* shows up in your mind and in your life. I think it will surprise you how it is hidden in plain view everywhere. Your worthiness has nothing to do with anything you *do*—it simply is what you *are*. That you are not worthy is a lie; you are worthy, most worthy of simple harmony in your body, mind, and spirit, simply because that is the essence of who and what you truly are.

LOVE, THE ULTIMATE HEALING TOOL

When I turned forty-one, my son Quinn said to me, "Next year you are going to be the answer to life, the universe, and everything!" He was referring to the fact that forty-two is the number that answers that question in the iconic book *The Hitchhiker's Guide to the Galaxy*. So when I turned forty-two, this was on my mind. It just so happened that at the time I was doing research on plasma and sacred geometry as an independent study for my master's degree, and so I was actually thinking about these subjects quite a lot.

One morning I was in Burlington having my car serviced and spent some time waiting and having breakfast in a café there. It suddenly came to me that I wanted to write, but I had no paper of any kind except for my appointment book. I opened up to the block schedule planner in the back and promptly wrote the poem below, putting each line in one of the boxes. I am not inclined to write poetry; in fact, I had quite a run-in with my sophomore English teacher in high school around poetry because I thought poems were silly and didn't want to have to write any, but this poem just sort of happened.

> I have figured out the answer to life, the universe, and
>   everything
> And it is . . .
> LOVE
> Love does make the world go 'round
> Gravity? Love
> Electricity? Love
> The strong force? Love
> The weak force? Love
> LOVE LOVE LOVE
> Could it be more simple?
> Could it be more obvious?
> But we don't see it
> Right in front of us
> All the time
> We don't see it
> We don't get it
> We are looking for something more
> But there is nothing more than
> LOVE
> Love is all there is
> Love is the driving force of the universe
> Of all creation
> Of physics
> Of biology
> Of metaphysics
> Pi = Love
> Phi = Love
> $E = mc^2 = love$
> It is all
> LOVE LOVE LOVE

Love is what heals you. Any place where you are not healed, you are not letting love happen in you, you are not loving yourself.

We have been taught that it is wrong to love ourselves, that it is selfish to love ourselves. It's okay and appropriate to love others, to have compassion for others, but not ourselves. This is a lie. This is why so many people are sick. We've been taught that it doesn't matter what we think or what we say, because we have no power. We believe we are powerless, because we do not understand the power of the word. We do not realize how creative words are.

One of the things I always say at lectures is that as a sound healer I have learned that the most powerful thing in the universe is right under your nose . . . and it's your mouth. By our words we create our lives.

What kinds of stories are you telling yourself and others about who you are? Healing is being willing to detach from your stories, to be willing to go into neutral and be open to other possibilities, to believe that you are worthy of those possibilities, to allow yourself to simply rest in the essence of the universe, which is, simply, love.

CONTINUING THE JOURNEY

Updated for Second Edition

It has now been twenty-four years since I first picked up a tuning fork, and ten years since I first started teaching what is now called Biofield Tuning. Our organization currently has eighteen teachers and over two thousand students and practitioners worldwide, and is poised to add many more by starting to offer virtual training. This is something we never believed was possible until we put it together and discovered that the work can actually be taught effectively in an online format.

What began as a blind fumble into unknown territory has opened up a whole new frontier, and I never cease to be amazed at how easily students pick up this subtle—and even strange—practice, and become proficient at it in a relatively short time. While it is very useful in many contexts, like anything, it definitely has its limitations and drawbacks. For one thing, it can be a bit exhausting when you first start learning it, and it takes time to build up the stamina to be able to conduct sessions all day long. As a practitioner, you have to keep yourself well rested, well fed, and in good balance in order to do the kind of energetic heavy lifting that this work requires.

Remember, you are working with resistance, sometimes very strong and deeply held resistance. The human mind is very powerful. Not only that, when you find an area of trauma in someone's biofield—and I have come across some extremely traumatic events in people's fields—the pathological oscillation in that area goes through your own body. You have to learn to feel it and then override it and ground it, and that takes some practice.

I have found that Biofield Tuning isn't very helpful as a stand-alone practice when disease has gone deeply into the body. For that reason we don't treat severe physical illness, or severe anything for that matter. It is very useful for mild to moderate issues of all kinds, and even better when combined with other practices such as bodywork and nutritional changes. Ultimately, I see it more as a tool for keeping people healthy and in balance rather than for pulling them back from the brink.

These days we have many different kinds of practitioners incorporating this work into what they are already doing with bodywork, chiropractic, Reiki, holistic nursing, acupuncture, and other forms of sound therapy. Even doctors, psychotherapists, and coaches have found this simple approach to be extremely useful with their patients and clients.

When I teach I encourage my students to find their own way to incorporate the two basic premises of sound balancing into their practice: combing, and using sound to find and balance areas of distortion in the field. Many people starting out in this technique get frustrated that they don't have the degree of immediate and precise intuition that I have developed over decades, which is why I always say, "Don't try to be me; figure out how to take this basic concept and use it to play to your own strengths and interests. Bring yourself to presence and be curious in your explorations of the biofield."

One thing that is slowly changing since I wrote my master's thesis back in 2011 is that while the biofield remains a battleground of sorts since we are still very much living in a world dominated by conventional medicine, a large amount of information is now surfacing that is demystifying "the energy in energy medicine," and many studies on the biofield have been published in the last decade, shining more light on the science behind many energy healing techniques. I have come to see this work as simple electricity (albeit a more subtle form of electricity that we don't fully understand yet), and increasingly I wonder why people even fuss about it as it seems so self-evident at this point.

The premise that this energy is actually electricity was the focus of a 2019 online forum, which I took part in, the Body Electric Summit. This event allowed me to present alongside thirty-five other researchers and providers who have all come to the same conclusion that I have: our bodies are electric. This electrical system is what comprises our biofield in its entirety—all of the electrical wiring and information flow in our bodies, as well as the wiring and flow of the magnetic field that surrounds the body.

This is who we are at a fundamental level, our inner light. When our light goes out, our body remains, but we ourself are gone. It is the health of this system (one could call it our mind in its totality, or even our soul or spirit) that is primary and gives rise to the chemical/ mechanical expressions of our body. When we successfully modulate and adjust our electrical system, we get right to the core of what's going on—our vibrational blueprint.

Biofield Tuning improves our electrical health by getting the noise and resistance out of our electrical system, and in this way, by rewiring us, clearing our habitual tangles and nonbeneficial patterns and restoring our original factory settings. Once we clear out the backlog of old emotions that are held in resistance (often creating inflammation in the body), we become much more resilient to current stressors, and it is easier to keep our energy and health up. It isn't so much about raising our vibration, but rather, clarifying our vibration, finding our vibrational sweet spot and raising the overall voltage of the battery that is our body.

My own personal journey with my own health and well-being through this work has been nothing short of amazing. I began receiving sessions from my first students in 2010, and immediately began to start clearing up the many health issues I had been suffering from, which I discovered were almost all a consequence of mismanaged emotions, lack of electrical grounding, poor boundaries, and repeating patterns from childhood.

At this point in 2021, I have personally received over five hundred Biofield Tuning sessions (including almost three hundred recorded group sessions that I conducted and put my own energy body into). At fifty-one years old, I have no health issues of any kind, huge amounts of energy, clarity, and focus, and the body I had as a teenager. Through creating tools and techniques with sound and teaching them to others, I have successfully lost twenty pounds, eliminated all digestive woes (stomachaches, heartburn, gas, bloating, indigestion, food allergies), gotten rid of chronic midback pain and knee pain, eliminated a colony of plantar warts on my feet, eliminated candida, overcome a decades-long sugar addiction, vastly improved my relationship with my husband, and much more. It wasn't for lack of trying that I had not improved these issues before 2010—it was because prior to that, I wasn't thinking electrically.

Each session you conduct and receive builds on the one before it, to bring greater clarity, lightness, and a sense of flow to your being. Each adjustment gets a bit of noise out of the signal and returns a bit of stuck light back into flow, raising the overall voltage of your system. I have witnessed thousands of people around me, students, clients, and friends, having this same experience. People become lighter, brighter, stronger, more free in their bodies and their minds, more liberated into their potential. They stop telling themselves stories of victimhood and lack, they start to take charge of the way they respond to life and loved ones, and their lives change, often dramatically, for the better.

When we move from thinking about taking care of our chemical and mechanical health to taking care of our electrical health, it's like discovering a backdoor hack that suddenly enables movement where there wasn't any previously. We discover rooms and dimensions that we suspected were within us but we didn't have access to, for in each of us are the codes for vibrant health, for living in harmony with nature and one another. These are our original factory settings. All we need do is be "in tune" to access them.

MOVING FORWARD

If you feel drawn to learning this work, you can start with something as simple as the Sonic Slider, which can be used on the body and in the field, on yourself or on others. You can also explore the basic premise of sound balancing with any instruments you may have—people have achieved similar results with singing bowls moved around the body, as well as with didgeridoos, the human voice, and more.

If you want to go deeper than that, I encourage you to try our Biofield Tuning toolkit, which has all the tools used by practitioners and over two hours of instructional videos. Acquiring this is the first step in becoming a practitioner, and it provides you with the information you need to work on family and friends. You can even use these tools as an addition to your current professional practice, but it's important to note that the toolkit and the instructional videos do not certify you as a Biofield Tuning practitioner, and do not give you permission to claim that you practice Biofield Tuning.

Another way to see if this method is right for you is to receive a session from one of our many practitioners worldwide, all of whom are trained to do the work, either in person or remotely. You can find a practitioner at our website, to receive a virtual session or an in-person session at our Burlington, Vermont, clinic. Please note: I strongly recommend that you commit to three sessions if possible, as many years of observation have shown me that while one can be very useful and even life-changing for many, the depth of transformation that can be achieved through a series is orders of magnitude beyond what can be achieved in just one session.

Another more affordable option is to try one of our live or recorded virtual group sessions. While the premise of recorded group tuning-fork healing sessions may sound a bit ridiculous (it certainly did to me before I tried it), early explorations of this medium of delivery (which was born of necessity due to the fact that my private practice had become too busy for me to see clients individually anymore) have provided us with ample evidence of its effectiveness. Many people have written to me and told me that they felt as if I was speaking directly to them and not a group, and reported that they felt energy moving in their bodies and experienced, in many cases, profound energetic shifts. Consequently, I went on to record hundreds of sessions, on just about every part of our physical and energetic body as possible. These sessions are a combination of coaching, education, and a Biofield Tuning adjustment, and as such they are all useful in deepening our understanding of the biofield and its anatomy and physiology.

Ultimately, this work leads us to a greater understanding of our own mind and body, and in this knowledge is found the power we need to improve our own health and well-being and help others, as well as our society as a whole. While I have done preliminary work in mapping the biofield and developing an effective method for the body to come back to its original energetic blueprint with a simple tuning fork, there is still so much more to be discovered! Biofield Tuning is a continually evolving and unfolding method focused on bringing the electric body into optimum health.

Wishing you all the best on your own journey of amplifying your inner light. Stay tuned!

Resources

www.biofieldtuning.com

www.biofieldtuningstore.com

www.biofieldtuningclinic.com

www.eileenmckusick.com

APPENDIX A

CASE STUDIES

Note: Names have been changed in this section.

Jim, age forty-seven, came to see me because he was having massive anxiety attacks whenever he had to drive somewhere, especially if it involved any kind of distance. He was also experiencing discomfort in his right shoulder and both heels. Jim was one of my more intriguing cases because when I began investigating his field I had the distinct impression of him being "off his rocker": his entire field had an oscillation in it, like a washing machine when it goes out of balance.

I found the edge of the oscillating field in each chakra and brought it to the midline of his body, where I had the curious and somewhat unusual perception of it "clicking" into place (most energy seems to either pool at the chakra or it feels like it is drawn inward to the body, but rarely ever clicks). I was particularly curious as to what his experience was after the session, and when he came to see me the following week he said, "I am completely cured. I had to go for a long drive the next day and it didn't bother me at all. The day after that I had to go for a longer drive and that didn't bother me at all either—in fact, I enjoyed it. And my shoulder and heel pain is also gone." When I checked in on his field I found that he had retained the balancing and was in very solid shape. He has maintained this and has not gone "off his rocker" again in the several years I have been seeing him once or twice a year for a general tune-up.

When Bill, age sixty, first came to see me, he was in terrible shape. He had suffered a string of terrible accidents, coming close to death in several of them. He had severe pain in his right hip, lower back, and left shoulder, was suffering from chronic and debilitating anxiety, had insomnia, and regularly experienced a major energy crash around three in the afternoon. He had tried acupuncture, chiropractic, massage, and osteopathic treatment, but nothing had helped more than just a little bit. And he refused to take painkillers.

Over the course of about eight or so sessions I was able to locate and neutralize the effects of each accident, even uncovering some that he had forgotten about. We got the anxiety to settle down, started getting him to sleep through the night, and eased his energy crashes in the afternoon. By the time we were through with this first round of sessions he was almost completely pain-free. Bill comes a few times a year now for a general tune-up.

The first time I saw Noreen, age twenty-two, was in a minisession I did at a health fair. These are seated sessions that last twenty to twenty-five minutes, and my approach is to ask the person if she has any problem areas with pain or tension, and then work solely on that, instead of going through the whole body. Though Noreen was young, she was already suffering from both rheumatoid arthritis and fibromyalgia. Her symptoms were so severe that she was unable to type her college papers and had to dictate them through dictation software.

Intuitively, I sensed that the origin of the issue was in her heart chakra, and sure enough, after just a moment or two of investigation, I found a large pocket of trapped energy in the left side of her heart from around the age of fourteen. She told me that was when the symptoms began. More investigation revealed that the issue was related to her relationship with her mother, which she confirmed. I was able to break up the stuck energy with relative ease and reintegrate it back into the heart chakra. Several days later I received an email from Noreen, telling me that she had gone home that evening and typed for three hours straight with no discomfort or pain in her hands or shoulders at all. We did a few more follow-up sessions, and she was able to cut way back on her medications and was able to maintain a much higher level of functioning with just occasional sessions after that.

Kristin, age thirty-two, signed up to do a series of ten sessions, more for emotional work than physical. One of Kristin's challenges in life had been her relationship with her father, who was a very difficult character. As a single mom, one of the things that Kristin had struggled with was finances, and while for the most part she had done a good job managing, there were times when she needed help. She was unwilling to ask her father for help because he always became quite upset, even though he had plenty of money and was in a position to help her out. The issue seemed to ignite the unresolved energies between the two of them.

A lot of the work we did involved clearing these energies, and during one particular session we uncovered and integrated a particularly charged area that had to do with money stuff between them from when she was a teenager. While we were engaged in these sessions, Kristin found a house that she really wanted to buy and wasn't sure how she was going to swing it, but was determined to figure it out. Out of the blue, the day after the session above, Kristin's father told her he would help her with the house, and he did, paying for it with cash—a completely out-of-character move on his part, especially since she had not asked him for help. But after the work we had done, it seemed the charge that had been between them on this subject was simply no longer there. Her relationship with him improved all around without her ever even having to discuss the subject with him.

Charlie, age sixty-five, came to me with no particular complaints but was curious about the work after he had seen his ex-wife have a powerful experience with it. One of the things that I was struck by was how stiff and unyielding the energy of his heart chakra was. It felt not only that he had hardened his heart emotionally, but that his physiology was also hardening along with it. After just a few sessions, Charlie found himself much better able to spontaneously communicate his feelings to his loved ones, allowing himself to feel the love and vulnerability that he had not allowed himself to feel for many years.

An artist, Charlie also returned to his first love, freehand drawing, a practice he had abandoned many years earlier to do computer-based artwork. He found himself with copious amounts of energy to draw from and became prolific, feeling like he was creating some of the best work he had ever done. He also experienced a diminishment in his arthritis pain.

Mickey, age twenty, had been put on Ritalin at age eight and had been on it throughout his teenage years. He had also turned to other drugs in his teens, was struggling with depression, and had tried unsuccessfully to get off all of the drugs. Mickey was the first person I ever worked on who had been on Ritalin for that long, and I was stunned to see the effect its long-term use had on his energy field. There were areas where there was simply a complete lack of any kind of energy at all, like his field was Swiss cheese. I was able to get these areas to fill in and balance, and after just a few sessions Mickey reported feeling less anxious, more clear, and more himself. He was able to get off the Ritalin, and in a short time he got off all the other drugs as well.

Fred, age thirty-two, came to me complaining of pain on the right side of his neck and the left side of his lower back. It had seemingly come out of nowhere, and he could not relate it to any injuries. He had been going to see a chiropractor, and the adjustments would help for a day or two, but then the pain would soon return. I discovered that his field was shifted strongly to the right side of his neck and the left side of his second chakra (frustration over not being heard), and learned that he had been fighting a lot with his girlfriend recently. I adjusted the energy and gave him some homework around dealing with the situation more effectively. When he returned the following week, he reported that he had not had any pain at all since he last saw me.

This was a classic case of psychosomatic pain: where it is the distortions in the energy body that give rise to the discomfort, not any particular pathology. This is the sort of issue that responds most profoundly to sound work, and is often untreatable by other means because it really is all in the person's mind, yet creates very real pain.

Phyllis, age forty-eight, came to see me because she was, in her words, "completely discombobulated." Phyllis's house had flooded completely the year before, forcing her to move to a temporary location while she and her husband cleaned up and restored the house, which they had to do while also running a business. As the year had worn on, Phyllis found herself more and more scattered and out of sorts and had been unable to get things back together by herself. After just three sessions, her energy level went way up, she was able to tackle projects she had not had the gumption to deal with, and was able to set better boundaries for herself at work and take the time off she needed. Phyllis actually ended up looking like a different person in the process of becoming more relaxed, centered, grounded, and coherent.

Matthew, age forty-four, came to me with no physical complaints but was in need of some deep emotional healing. He had been adopted into a family that had treated him very cruelly and had struggled with severe dyslexia that prevented him from learning to read until he was thirteen. His adoptive family had been very intolerant of his disability and had routinely punished him for it, driving him into a deep depression. To make matters worse, he had connected with his birth mother when he was twenty-one and was welcomed into her new family for a time, only to be suddenly and inexplicably cast out again. Matthew had struggled through one relationship after another but continually felt as if his soul was being sucked out of him by the women in his life.

I was able to locate some significant tears in the edge of his field on the left side, in areas relating to sadness, mother, and frustration—

places where he had been both leaking energy and attracting people who were more than willing to take it from him. Early trauma around mother, such as what Matthew had experienced in being adopted, and then his subsequent lack of chemistry with his adoptive mother, had created wounds that remained raw throughout his lifetime. With sound we were able to locate and heal these vibrational disruptions.

We had to do a fair number of sessions to counter all of the non-beneficial influences in his life, but he found himself feeling more and more centered and emotionally free and better able to express himself creatively. He began to feel as if he really was worthy and had something to offer the world, and was able to formulate a vocation for himself that was supportive of this new perspective. He recently informed me that he had a new partner and it was a relationship that was completely different from any he had previously, and far more nurturing.

Andrew, age thirty-two, came to me in terrible shape—exhausted, stressed, and burned out. Andrew owned his own business and was a victim of his own success. He worked long hours, often had tight dead-lines, and had a difficult employee who was a continual source of stress. He had grown up with an abusive alcoholic father who had also been the child of an abusive alcoholic father, and so his childhood had been fraught with nonstop acute stress.

Because I most often start on the left side of the body, in our first session together I came across the signal from Andrew's left adrenal before I came across the signal from his right one. It was, far and away, the most dissonant adrenal I'd ever heard, and I said to him, "If your left adrenal sounds this bad (because most people's right adre-nals are more activated and "out" than their left), I can't even imagine what your right one is going to sound like." Sure enough, when I got over to his right side, I listened for the rhythm of that adrenal and found nothing. Energetically, it felt like pudding, and had clearly been pushed so far that it had actually gone completely offline. It was no wonder he was finding it harder and harder to handle the stress in his life. Over the course of about six sessions, I resurrected and balanced Andrew's adrenals and helped restore wholeness and balance to his fairly shattered and tattered field. His life subsequently underwent a radical transformation. He sold his business and his house and moved to a different climate, where he got a job that he loved, working for someone else, and he was able to create a life that was no longer full of chronic stress.

TESTIMONIALS FROM MY STUDENTS

While I was working on the sixth chakra to the right, I could hear music faintly in the background, and it got louder over a period of a minute, and so I stopped, commenting to my client that I could clearly hear carnival/circus music. (I thought it was just in my head but it was so prevalent that I had to say something.) And the client remarked that at that moment she was thinking about how crazy her life is, and that it's like a circus, and she was constructing the whole circus in her mind while I was hearing the music, so this could be a case of psychic music.

ADAM MEACHEM

I have decided to focus on the sound healing arts after working with Eileen. What convinced me to continue was the positive effects I have been able to produce on the people I have worked with. I have also seen great improvement in my own health and well-being from receiving sessions.

MARY BETH GIROUX

I'm a certified Reiki master, Karuna master, and magnified healer, but I was looking for more. My husband bought me a singing bowl, and I found a bowl class and became certified. It has been so wonderful, and I realized it was sound I had to work with. I then took a fork class but was still looking for more, and that's when I found Eileen. I saw her video and called her. She was so insightful and gave me a book to read. I found a way to make it to her to take class 1 on Biofield Tuning. This is what I had been looking for.

The reaction I'm getting has been better that I imagined. Something new always comes about and teaches me something. The people I have treated with tuning forks never cease to amaze me. Some have cried through the treatment and then told me later they felt so relieved and relaxed. People had allergies and couldn't breathe well and this also made them feel better. I worked on a woman's throat chakra and it swelled up at first but the outcome was great. She spoke up and things started working out the way she needed them to. The list goes on, and the people I have been working on are now looking for more treatments. I can't begin to say how grateful I am to be able to help people through the use of sound.

DEBRA DION

There's something deeply familiar about using the tuning forks and the process of relating to and connecting with people. I think that's because of two things: my background as a musician and a dancer, and my background in mediation and conflict resolution.

As a musician and dancer, I feel comfortable and enjoy being in the world of vibration, and I also enjoy working spatially with human beings. However, because it was initially pretty easy to "feel" the vibrations, it wasn't as easy for me to "hear" the changes in the forks, especially as I worked with higher notes. As I practice, though, I find I am having breakthroughs in hearing; I couldn't distinguish under- and overtone notes initially, and now I can. I've learned as much being a practice body for others as I have as a practitioner. When there is no pressure on me to actually do anything, I find I can more easily focus my attention. I'm sure there's more to hear, and I look forward to those breakthroughs too.

Also—I feel comfortable in the realm of listening deeply to people talk about what comes up for them in the process. I think one of the gifts that I bring from my background and training in mediation (and somehow, also, just from my "being") is a strong sense of listening deeply, trusting my own intuition and the ability to check out that intuition gracefully, and being client-centered. I can easily shift between what I'm hearing/feeling/intuiting to doing reflective listening (and now "sponge listening"!) and creative inquiry to support whatever's coming up for the client.

K. M.

Biofield Tuning has changed my life. I originally tried it because I was told by other therapists that it had been a very beneficial and profound experience for them. I was going through a time of crisis in my life. I cried though the whole first session. I felt like Eileen hit the nail on the head in every aspect of my life where I felt pain. It was a huge relief and release of pent-up emotion. Afterward, I felt like I was in an altered state. The tears kept pouring out of my eyes even though I had no idea why. I felt lighter and calmer and more peaceful.

Further sessions were less intense but no less profound. I continued receiving sessions with Eileen as often as possible, sometimes once a week, sometimes once a month. It helped me through the intensity I was experiencing at the time and continues to be a source of healing and health for me.

I began studying sound therapy in Eileen's pilot class. Learning Biofield Tuning has taught me how to listen to my intuition. I've realized that we are all intuitive; we only need to "tune in" to hear it. Now I have a new depth in my professional healing practice. I use the forks alone in sound therapy sessions, in my massage sessions, and as first aid. I find the vibrations of the forks to be like a sonic massage of body, emotions, and mind. I am so glad to have Biofield Tuning in my life as a healing tool for others and myself.

CARA JOY

I am realizing in this work how, ultimately, it is the forks themselves that are doing the work, not me—I am more the guide in a way, and I can trust that the forks will do their work, even as I am still very much a beginner. I just had a friend with adrenal issues tell me that while she didn't feel much during our second session, afterward she felt this rush of energy like she hadn't felt in a very long time, and it reminded her what it felt like to have energy and feel good again. It only lasted several hours and then her exhaustion set in again, but she said it helped just to feel what that was like and know it was possible. I hadn't been sure I'd done a whole lot since she didn't seem to feel things the way she did the first time. After she told me this I had the "aha" moment that the forks are going to have some kind of effect on people regardless of my abilities. This realization has made me more aware of, and more respectful of, the potential power (both healing and, if used in ignorance or carelessly, harmful) of the forks, and so to be extravigilant about follow-up with people.

SUSANNAH BLACHLY

For four years I have worked with Eileen personally with Biofield Tuning. When I first began I found that my body took in the vibrations of the tuning forks like a sponge. The pain I experienced at the time was greatly relieved. I felt better and better over the course of treatment over two years, and my stress level was always significantly diminished after a session.

I am an artist and trained in the Netherlands in painting therapy. About fifteen years ago I purchased two tuning forks, and I really didn't know what to do with them. Nearly two years ago I was asked to go to the hospital to work with a patient with depression who had tried to commit suicide. Intuitively, along with my color box of paints, I took my tuning forks. The patient responded so well to the tuning forks that I decided I owed it to that person to take the training with Eileen.

After beginning my training, when I was working on this patient with sound, when placing the vibrating fork on the foot, there was no sensation of vibration past a few toes closest to the fork. Now this person can feel the whole foot vibrating. This person continues to do both therapeutic modalities and is becoming more and more successful in raking up a healthy lifestyle and is now able to stand on their own two feet. To be sure, these two modalities are working well in tandem.

MARTHA LOVING

I, for some unknown reason, was attracted to taking Eileen's class. I had a single tuning fork from a special Native American friend of mine but didn't really know how to use it to benefit anyone. I saw Eileen's class posted and decided to give it a whirl. I loved the class and was noticing how people were responding to the forks, some in a very dramatic way. I practiced Reiki but never had gotten that kind of response. I felt the sound went much deeper into the field.

I then decided maybe I should go to a session with Eileen. Well, I have never, ever experienced anything so profound in my entire life! I felt like a whole lifetime of bottled up shit (excuse my profanity) came out of that session. I came to the awesome conclusion that I need to save myself first then take care of others. I have steadily felt like I've been coming into my own power source in a balanced way. I'm healthier from the inside out. I'm truly grateful for this healing tool that came into my life. I can both hear and feel when I'm coming up against resistance in a person's biofield when I am practicing with the forks. Both I and some people I have worked on have heard it get very loud in some places—very interesting. I've also had people say they can feel if I'm twisting or manipulating the forks without them seeing me doing this.

ROBIN FARRAR

I was fascinated the first time I went to see Eileen to experience the tuning forks. I could hear the disturbance of sound in my energy field and was amazed by the questions she asked me about my experiences in the past. I knew I wanted to learn how to do it. I am a homeopathic and Heilkunst practitioner so I am used to using energy, but in a much more specific form.

Homeopathy and Heilkunst, an entire system of medicine based on homeopathy, are intellectual and intuitive processes that look at one's pain to find the appropriate homeopathic remedies and nutritional support to resolve both the physical and emotional issues. To find the appropriate remedies I ask a lot of questions, such as what was happening when the symptoms started, what makes it better and worse, time of day when it's more of a problem, etc. Many people don't know the answers. They are not aware of themselves enough to give me the information, so I can look up the symptoms in the materia medica.

Sound therapy utilizes the practitioner's gamut, or inner wisdom, to feel the dissonance in an energy field. As the client feels or hears the dissonance, the practitioner bears witness so the client can allow the healing frequencies to dissolve the stuck pain. That experience can then be integrated so they can move forward with greater clarity.

I have been amazed at how different people experience the tuning forks. Some people hear the sound changes, others feel pressure or tingling, some feel an intensity of pain and then it is gone. People are able to laugh at situations that have been so painful to them and realize that they have options. People have been able to remember situations just by hearing or feeling the energy changing in their bodies or the sound dissonance. Headaches, anxiety, panic attacks, TMJ, back tension, knee issues, and herpes outbreaks have been lessened or dissipated totally. I use the weighted forks on people when they come for a homeopathic session and use them for physical pain as well, and have them use the forks on themselves while I am making up remedies for them. I have found it an invaluable addition to my practice.

JUDY JARVIS

Like the art of massage, anyone can grasp the basics of Biofield Tuning if they have an interest in the material. But it takes a sensitivity to wield these forks with true power, and an awareness of slight differentiations in sound, or the ability to feel shifts in energetics that come through the fork as you hold it in your hand. Both of these can be fostered in anyone who is drawn to using this balancing modality.

When I am working with the forks I am very aware of the tone and pitch, the overtones and undertones. When I land on a discrepancy in the field, the sound will sharpen or dim, the overtones and undertones may increase or disappear. This signals me to combine this sensory input with any one of the numerous techniques that Eileen has taught me to return the tone to its original pitch. When I am receiving Biofield Tuning work and this occurs, the use of the fork on my biofield is very noticeable. I can actually feel the sound vibration—and have been known to laugh or cry, as a natural reaction to the repair that is occurring.

I know this method works because I have been on the giving and the receiving end of numerous healing and balancing experiences. I feel blessed to have had the privilege to work with Eileen and learn her self-created technique directly. It would not be an understatement to say that the last year and a half spent studying tuning forks with Eileen McKusick has been some of the most transformational time of my life.

ASHLEY LAUX

CHAKRA TABLES AND BIOFIELD ANATOMY MAPS

MINOR CHAKRAS

CHAKRA	TUNING FORK	RELATES TO	LEFT IMBALANCE	RIGHT IMBALANCE	GENERAL INDICATION
Feet	UT/C	potential link to past lives	undefined	undefined	ability to support oneself and take the next steps in life
Knees	UT/C	degree of inner and outer freedom	left knee: things from the past that are no longer indicated or appropriate in the present	right knee: challenges moving forward; obstacles within or without; slow or complicated birth experience	front of knees: "greener-pasture" thinking

MAJOR CHAKRAS

CHAKRA/ PLEXUS	COLOR	SOLFEGGIO FORK/ HARMONIC FORK	GOVERNS	RELATES TO	LEFT IMBALANCE	RIGHT IMBALANCE	OVERALL LOW ENERGY	HEALTHY
Root/ First	red	UT/C	tailbone, relation to ground, legs and feet, hip joints, pelvis	home life, security, tribe, right livelihood, rootedness, groundedness	not doing, indolence, thinking about doing but not doing, no rubber on the road—no connection between thoughts and actions	overly active physically— doing too much, overly active mentally— thinking too much, often guilt driven	low energy, not sleeping well, not well rested, fighting infection	thoughts and feelings in accordance with actions, present in the now, comfortable in home, right livelihood, high energy level
Sacral/ Second	orange	RE/D	reproductive organs, bladder, large intestine, small intestine	sexuality, creativity, cash flow, self-worth, intimate relationships	frustration, disappointment	guilt, shame	creatively stuck, unhealthy intimate relationships, low self-worth	healthy intimate relationships, creatively flowing

Chakra	Color	Note	Location	Governs			Underactive	Balanced
Solar Plexus/ Third	yellow	MI/E	spleen, pancreas, stomach, kidneys, adrenals, liver, gallbladder, and relationship with father and mother	self-confidence, self-esteem, how we interface with others' energies, setting goals and achieving them	powerlessness	anger	not assertive, challenged by setting and achieving goals, easily overwhelmed by others' energy	assertive, able to advocate for self, able to complete projects
Heart/ Fourth	green	FA/F	heart, lungs	giving and receiving love, compassion, and gratitude	sadness, grief, and loss	saying yes when we mean no, overdoing for others	challenge to give and receive love, harboring old pain, suffering from depression	following heart's desires, able to love freely
Throat/ Fifth	blue	SOL/G	thyroid, jaw, throat, faculty of hearing	communication, speaking our truth, creativity	not communicating or expressing, holding back	speaking and not being heard	not expressing self, thyroid issues, holding back	communicating clearly, being heard, particularly strong energy relates to teacher, writer, or other communication vocation

MAJOR CHAKRAS (continued)

CHAKRA/ PLEXUS	COLOR	SOLFEGGIO FORK/ HARMONIC FORK	GOVERNS	RELATES TO	LEFT IMBALANCE	RIGHT IMBALANCE	OVERALL LOW ENERGY	HEALTHY
Third Eye/ Sixth	purple or indigo	LA/A	pineal gland, brain	intuition, thought processes	worrying about the future	overthinking about the past	inability to focus, distrust or disconnection from intuition	clear third eye perception, mental focus and acuity
Crown/ Seventh	white or purple	963 Hz/B	brain, relationship with time, relationship with the Divine	higher thinking, spatial intelligence, music	undefined	undefined	difficulty focusing, overwhelmed by life, often a consequence of too much time inside, especially under fluorescent lights	right relationship with time and the Divine, aided by plenty of time outside

BIOFIELD ANATOMY ENERGETIC IMBALANCES

Front view

Right side: Masculine side

Left side: Feminine side

Not enough time;
disconnect from nature

Thinking about the past

Worrying about the future

Speaking but not being heard

That which we do not express

Saying yes when we mean
no; emotional caretaking

Sadness; grief; loss

Relationship with father;
anger

Relationship with mother;
powerlessness

Guilt; shame

Frustration; resentment

Busyness; overdoing

Things we want to be
doing but are not doing

Challenges moving forward;
confusion; obstacles

Challenges letting go;
discomfort with change

BIOFIELD ANATOMY ENERGETIC IMBALANCES

Back view

Areas of discomfort or pain and their associated imbalances are noted

Left side: Feminine side

Right side: Masculine side

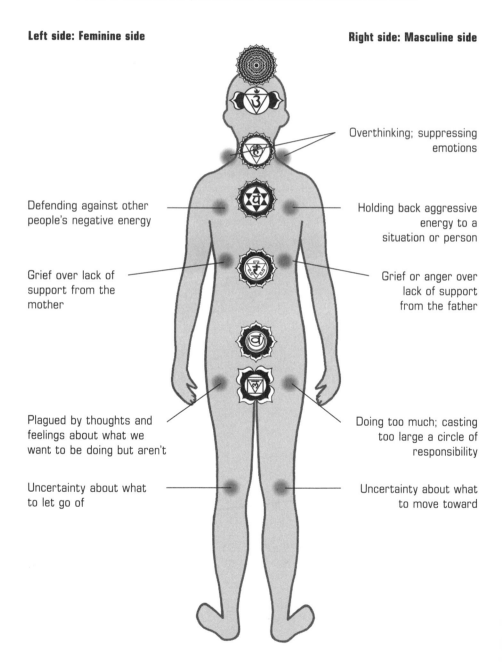

Overthinking; suppressing emotions

Defending against other people's negative energy

Holding back aggressive energy to a situation or person

Grief over lack of support from the mother

Grief or anger over lack of support from the father

Plagued by thoughts and feelings about what we want to be doing but aren't

Doing too much; casting too large a circle of responsibility

Uncertainty about what to let go of

Uncertainty about what to move toward

NOTES

FOREWORD

1. Becker and Selden, *Body Electric.*
2. Szent-Györgyi, *Bioenergetics.*
3. Pollack, *Fourth Phase.*
4. Oschman, *Energy Medicine;* Albrecht-Buehler, "In Defense."
5. Markov, "Biological Windows."
6. Del Giudice, Spinetti, and Tedeschi, "Water Dynamics."
7. Fröhlich, "Long-Range Coherence."
8. Fleming, "Electromagnetic Self-Field Theory."
9. Bauer, Cooper, and Fleming, "Effects."
10. Rauscher, "Quantum Mechanics."
11. Reid, "Special Relationship."
12. Del Giudice, Spinetti, and Tedeschi, "Water Dynamics"; Pollack, *Fourth Phase.*
13. Pall, "Biomagnetic Fields."

INTRODUCTION. TRUTH HAS 144 SIDES

1. Anderson, "Emerging Science," 1.
2. Gary Schwartz, "True versus Pseudo-Skepticism," Dr. Gary Schwartz (website, site discontinued).
3. Dunning, "Facts and Fiction."
4. Rosch, "Reminiscenses."

247

1. THE POWER OF WORDS

1. Carey, "Princeton Lab."

2. Patton, *Utilization-Focused Evaluation,* 203.

3. Higgo, "A Lazy Layman's Guide to Quantum Physics."

2. SOUND—WHAT IS IT?

1. Tennenbaum, "Foundations."

2. Moore, "Use of a Tuning Fork."

3. Lipton, *Biology,* 53.

4. USING SOUND THERAPEUTICALLY

1. Hadjiargyrou, McLeod, Ryaby, and Rubin, "Enhancement of Fracture Healing."

2. Srbely and Dickey, "Randomized Controlled Study."

3. Byl, "Use of Ultrasound."

4. Wilkins, "Magnetic Resonance."

5. Silber, "Bars."

6. Taylor, "Biomedical Theory."

7. Kim, et al., "Emotional, Motivational, and Interpersonal."

8. Chanda and Levitin, "Neurochemistry," 187.

9. Freeman, *Mosby's,* 21.

10. Boyd-Brewer, "Vibroacoustic Therapy."

11. Boyd-Brewer, "Vibroacoustic Therapy."

12. Edelson, et al., "Auditory Integration."

13. Lazar, et al., "Functional Brain Mapping."

14. Kreutz, et al., "Effects of Choir Singing."

15. Salaman, et al., "Sound Therapy," RA119.

16. Wahbeh, et al., "Binaural Beat."

17. Lynes, *Cancer Cure.*

5. WIDENING MY UNDERSTANDING OF PLASMA AND AETHER

1. Alvino, "The Human Energy Field."

2. Brennan, *Hands of Light.*

3. McCraty, et al., "Resonant Heart," 16.

4. Martin, "Discover the Ultimate Power of Your Heart," Finerminds (website, article no longer available), 2009.

5. Friedlander, *Golden Wand,* 83.

6. Einstein, *Sidelights,* 23.

6. DISCOVERING THE BIOFIELD IN SCIENCE

1. Oschman, *Energy Medicine,* 8.

2. Oschman, *Energy Medicine,* 5.

3. Oschman, *Energy Medicine,* 5.

4. Oschman, *Energy Medicine,* 5.

5. Sheldrake, "FAQs: What are the morphic fields? How do they fit into your hypothesis of formative causation?" Rupert Sheldrake (website).

6. Sheldrake, "FAQs: What do you think the repercussions would be if your Hypothesis of Formative Causation were to be vindicated?" Rupert Sheldrake (website).

7. Rubik, "Biofield Hypothesis," 713.

8. Rubik, "Biofield Hypothesis," 713.

9. Tiller, *Science and Human Transformation.*

10. "Research," Valerie V. Hunt (website).

11. Hunt, *Infinite Mind.*

12. Swanson, *Life Force.*

13. Swanson, *Life Force.*

14. Oschman, *Energy Medicine.*

15. Swanson, *Life Force.*

16. Swanson, *Life Force.*

17. Swanson, *Life Force.*

18. Swanson, *Life Force.*

19. Swanson, *Life Force.*

20. Gilman, "Memory."

21. Swanson, *Life Force.*

22. Pert, *Molecules of Emotion.*

23. Stenger, "Bioenergetic Fields."

24. Nelson and Schwartz, "Human Biofield," 93.

25. Schwartz, *Energy Healings.*

7. THE ANATOMY OF THE BIOFIELD

1. Sol Luckman, personal email communication, March 22, 2013.

2. Sarkar, "Consciousness—Our Third Eye," LifePositive.

9. BIOFIELD ANATOMY WISDOM

1. Pert, *Molecules.*

BIBLIOGRAPHY

Albrecht-Buehler, Guenter. "In Defense of 'Nonmolecular' Biology." *International Review of Cytology* 120, (1990): 191–242.

Alfred, Jay. *Our Invisible Bodies: Scientific Evidence for Subtle Bodies.* Indiana: Trafford, 2006.

Alvino, Gloria. "The Human Energy Field in Relation to Science, Consciousness, and Health." The VXM Network (website). 1996.

Anderson, John, and Larry Trivieri, eds. *Alternative Medicine: The Definitive Guide,* 2nd ed. Berkeley, Calif.: Celestial Arts, 2002.

Anderson, Scott Virdin. "The Emerging Science of Subtle Energy." *The Noetic Post* 1, no. 2 (Spring/Summer 2010): 1–3.

Bauer, E. B., K. Cooper, and A. H. J. Fleming. "The Effects of Acoustic Frequencies on Core Tendon Lesions of the Thoroughbred Racehorse." *BEMS* 27 (June 19–25, 2005).

Beck, Martha. *Expecting Adam: A True Story of Birth, Transformation and Unconditional Love.* New York: Berkley Books, 2000.

Becker, Robert, and Gary Selden. *The Body Electric: Electromagnetism and the Foundation of Life.* New York: William Morrow, 1998.

Berbari, Nicholas F., Amber K. O'Connor, Courtney J. Haycraft, and Bradley K. Yoder. "The Primary Cilium as a Complex Signaling Center." *Current Biology* 19, no. 13 (2009): R526–35.

Boyd-Brewer, Chris. "Vibroacoustic Therapy: Sound Vibrations in Medicine." *Alternative and Complementary Therapies* 9, no. 5 (2004): 257–63.

Brennan, Barbara. *Hands of Light: A Guide to Healing through the Human Energy Field.* New York: Bantam, 1988.

Buchanan, Gary Robert. *SONA: Healing with Wave Front BIOresonance.* Reno, Nev.: International Community Guilds, 2008.

Byl, Nancy N. "The Use of Ultrasound as an Enhancer for Transcutaneous Drug Delivery: Phonophoresis." *Journal of the American Physical Therapy Association* 75, no. 6 (1995): 539–53.

Capps, Charles. *The Tongue: A Creative Force.* England, Ark.: Capps Publishing, 1976.

Carey, Benedict. "A Princeton Lab on ESP Plans to Close Its Doors," *New York Times* (online), February 10, 2007.

Chanda, Mona Lisa, and Daniel J. Levitin. "The Neurochemistry of Music." *Trends in Cognitive Sciences* 17, no. 4 (2013): 179–93.

Clandinin, D. Jean, ed. *Handbook of Narrative Inquiry: Mapping a Methodology.* Thousand Oaks, Calif.: Sage Publications, 2007.

Clandinin, D. Jean and Michael Connelly. *Narrative Inquiry: Experience and Story in Qualitative Research.* San Francisco, Calif.: Jossey-Bass, 2000.

Cousineau, Denis. "The Rise of Quantitative Methods of Psychology." *Tutorial in Quantitatitve Methods for Psychology* 1, no. 1 (2005): 1–3.

Del Giudice, E., P. R. Spinetti, and A. Tedeschi. "Water Dynamics at the Root of Metamorphosis in Living Organisms." *Water* 2, no. 3 (2010): 566–86.

Dunning, Brian. "Facts and Fiction of the Schumann Resonance." *Skeptoid,* podcast 352.

Edelson, Stephen M., Deborah Arin, Margaret Bauman, Scott E. Lukas, Jane H. Rudy, Michelle Sholar, Bernard Rimland. "Auditory Integration Training: A Double-Blind Study of Behavioral and Electrophysiological Effects in People with Autism." *Focus on Autism and Other Developmental Disabilities* 14, no. 2 (June 1999): 73–81.

Einstein, Albert. *Sidelights on Relativity.* Elegant Ebooks, ibiblio (website).

Emoto, Masuru. *The Hidden Messages in Water.* Hillsboro, Ore.: Beyond Words Publishing, 2004.

Fleming, A. H. J. "Electromagnetic Self-Field Theory and Its Application to the Hydrogen Atom." *Physics Essays* 18, no. 3 (2005): 265–85.

Freeman, Lyn. *Mosby's Complementary and Alternative Medicine: A Research-Based Approach,* 3rd ed. St. Louis, Mo.: Mosby's Inc., 2008.

Friedlander, Walter J. *The Golden Wand of Medicine: A History of the Caduceus Symbol in Medicine.* Westport, Conn.: Greenwood Press, 1992.

Fröhlich, H. "Long-Range Coherence and Energy Storage in Biological Systems." *International Journal of Quantum Chemistry* 2, no. 5 (1968): 641–49.

Gaynor, Mitchell L. *The Healing Power of Sound: Recovery from Life-Threatening Illness Using Sound, Voice, and Music.* Boston: Shambhala, 2002.

Gilman, R. "Memory and Morphogenetic Fields." *In Context* 6 (Summer 1984): 11.

Hadjiargyrou, Michael, Kenneth McLeod, John P. Ryaby, and Clinton Rubin. "Enhancement of Fracture Healing by Low Intensity Ultrasound." *Clinical Orthopaedics and Related Research* 355 (1998): 216–29.

Hawkins, David. *Power vs Force: The Hidden Determinants of Human Behavior,* rev. ed. Hay House, 2012.

Higgo, James. "A Lazy Layman's Guide to Quantum Physics." SCRIBD (website).

Horowitz, Leonard G., and Joseph S. Pulco. *Healing Codes for the Biological Apocalypse.* Tetrahedron Publishing, 2001.

Hunt, Valerie. *Infinite Mind: Science of the Human Vibrations of Consciousness.* Malibu, Calif.: Malibu Publishing, 1996.

Jain, Shamini, and Paul Mills. "Biofield Therapies: Helpful or Full of Hype? A Best Evidence Synthesis." *International Journal of Behavioral Medicine* 17, no. 1 (2010): 1–16.

Kim, Jinah, Tony Wigram, and Christian Gold. "Emotional, Motivational, and Interpersonal Responsiveness of Children with Autism in Improvisational Music Therapy." *Austism* 13 (2009): 389–409.

Kreutz, Gunter, Stephan Bongard, Sonja Rohrmann, Volker Hodapp, and Dorothee Grebe. "Effects of Choir Singing and Listening on Secretory Immunoglobulin A, Cortisol, and Emotional State." *Journal of Behavioral Medicine* 27, no. 6 (December 2004): 623–35.

Kuhn, Thomas S. *The Structure of Scientific Revolutions,* 3rd ed. Chicago: University of Chicago Press, 1996.

LaViolette, Paul A. *Secrets of Antigravity Propulsion: Tesla, UFOs, and Classified Aerospace Technology.* Rochester, Vt.: Bear & Co., 2008.

Lazar, Sara W., George Bush, Randy L. Gollub, Gregory L. Fricchione, Gurucharan Khalsa, and Herbert Benson. "Functional Brain Mapping of the Relaxation Response and Meditation." *NeuroReport* 11, no. 7 (2000): 1581–85.

Levitin, Daniel J. *This Is Your Brain on Music.* New York: Plume/Penguin, 2007.

Lipton, Bruce H. *The Biology of Belief: Unleashing the Power of Consciousness, Matter, and Miracles.* New York: Hay House, 2005.

Lockhart, Maureen. *The Subtle Energy Body: The Complete Guide.* Rochester, Vt.: Inner Traditions, 2010.

Luckman, Sol. *Conscious Healing: Book One of the Regenetics Method.* Raleigh, N.C.: Crow Rising, 2010.

———. *Potentiate Your DNA: A Practical Guide to Healing and Transformation with the Regenetics Method.* Raleigh, N.C.: Crow Rising, 2011.

Lynes, Barry. *The Cancer Cure That Worked: 50 Years of Suppression.* South Lake Tahoe, Calif.: BioMed Publishing Group, 1987.

Markov, Marko S. "'Biological Windows': A Tribute to W. Ross Adey." *Environmentalist* 25, no. 2–4, (2005): 67–74.

Mason, Russ. "The Sound Medicine of Brian Dailey, M.D., F.A.C.E.P." *Alternative and Complementary Therapies* 10, no. 3 (June 2004): 156–60.

McCraty, Rollin, Raymond Trevor Bradley, and Dana Tomasino. "The Resonant Heart." *Ions Shift* 5 (December 2004–February 2005): 15–19.

Moore, Michael Bryan. "The Use of a Tuning Fork and Stethoscope to Identify Fractures." *Journal of Athletic Training* 44, no. 3 (2009): 272–74.

Myss, Carolyn. *Anatomy of the Spirit: The Seven Stages of Power and Healing.* New York: Harmony, 1997.

Nelson, Lonnie, A., and Gary E. Schwartz. "Human Biofield and Intention Detection: Individual Differences." *Journal of Alternative and Complementary Medicine* 11, no. 1 (2005): 93–101.

Oschman, James. *Energy Medicine: The Scientific Basis.* New York: Churchill Livingstone, 2000.

Pall, Martin L. "Biomagnetic Fields Act via Activation of Voltage-Gated Calcium Channels to Produce Beneficial or Adverse Effects." *Journal of Cellular and Molecular Medicine* 17, no. 8 (2013): 958–65.

Patton, Michael Quinn. *Utilization-Focused Evaluation,* 4th ed. Beverly Hills, Calif.: Sage Publications, 2008.

Pert, Candace. *Molecules of Emotion: The Science behind Mind-Body Medicine.* New York: Simon and Schuster, 1999.

Pollack, Gerald. *The Fourth Phase of Water: Beyond Solid, Liquid, and Vapor.* Seattle, Wash.: Ebner & Sons, 2013.

Rapport, Frances, ed. *New Qualitative Methodologies in Health and Social Research.* New York/London: Routledge, 2004.

Rauscher, E.A. "Quantum Mechanics and the Role for Consciousness in the Physical World." *Subtle Energy and Energy Medicine* 16, no. 1 (2006): 1–42.

Reid, John S. "The Special Relationship between Sound and Light, with Implications for Sound and Light Therapy." *Subtle Energy and Energy Medicine* 17, no. 3 (2007): 215–31.

Robertson, Valma J., and Kerry G. Baker. "A Review of Therapeutic Ultrasound: Effectiveness Studies." *Physical Therapy* 81, no. 7 (2001): 1339–50.

Rosch, Paul John. "Reminiscenses of Hans Seyle and the Birth of Stress." *International Journal of Emerging Mental Health* 1, no. 1 (1999): 59–66.

Rubik, Beverly. "The Biofield Hypothesis: Its Biophysical Basis and Role in Medicine." *Journal of Alternative and Complementary Medicine* 8, no. 6 (2002): 703–17.

Salaman, Elliott, Minsun Kim, John Beaulieu, and Geroge B. Stefano. "Sound Therapy Induced Relaxation: Down Regulating Stress

Processes and Pathologies." *Medical Science Monitor* 9, no. 5 (2003): RA116–21.

Schwartz, Gary. *The Energy Healing Experiments: Science Reveals Our Natural Power to Heal.* New York: Atria, 2008.

Scott, Donald. *The Electric Sky.* Portland, Ore.: Mikamar Publishing, 2006.

Sheldrake, Rupert. *The Presence of the Past: Morphic Resonance and the Memory of Nature,* 4th ed. Rochester, Vt.: Park Street Press, 2012.

Silber, Laya. "Bars behind Bars: The Impact of a Women's Prison Choir on Social Harmony." *Music Education Research* 7, no. 2 (2005): 251–71.

Srbely, John Z., and James P. Dickey. "Randomized Controlled Study of the Antinociceptive Effect of Ultrasound on Trigger Point Sensitivity: Novel Applications in Myofascial Therapy." *Clinical Rehabilitation* 21, no. 5 (2007): 411–17.

Stenger, Victor. "Bioenergetic Fields." *Scientific Review of Alternative Medicine* 3, no. 1 (1999): 16–21.

Swanson, Claude. *Life Force, the Scientific Basis: Breakthrough Physics of Energy Medicine, Healing, Chi and Quantum Consciousness.* Tucson, Ariz.: Poseidia Press, 2009.

Szent-Györgyi, Albert. *Bioenergetics.* New York: Academic Press, 1957.

Tarnis, Richard, and Dean Radin. "The Timing of Paradigm Shifts." *Noetic Now* 18 (2012).

Taylor, D. B. "The Biomedical Theory of Music Therapy." In *Introduction to Approaches in Music Therapy,* 2nd ed., edited by Alice-Ann Darrow, 105–27. Silver Spring, Md.: American Music Therapy Association, 2008.

Tennenbaum, Jonathan. "The Foundations of Scientific Musical Tuning." *Fidelio* 1, no. 1 (1991–92).

Tompkins, Peter. *The Secret Life of Plants: A Fascinating Account of the Physical, Emotional, and Spiritual Relations between Plants and Man.* New York: Harper and Row, 1989.

Tiller, William. *Science and Human Transformation: Subtle Energies, Consciousness and Intention.* Walnut Creek, Calif.: Pavior, 1997.

Wahbeh, H., C. Calabrese, and H. Zwickey. "Binaural Beat Technology in Humans: A Pilot Study to Assess Psychologic and Physiologic Effects." *Journal of Alternative and Complementary Medicine* 13, no. 1 (Jan–Feb 2007): 25–32.

Wilkins, S. "Magnetic Resonance-Guided Focused Ultrasound Overview." *Journal of Radiology* 18 (2007): 132–38.

Witte, Darlene. *Adult Memories of Childhood Play Experiences: Emergence of Metaphoric Themes.* Edmonton, AB: University of Alberta, 1989.

INDEX

Page numbers in *italics* refer to illustrations.